T5-CVG-222

NURSING HOME LIFE:
What It Is and What It Could Be

Clifford Bennett, Ph.D.

The Tiresias Press, Inc., New York City

Dedication

To my late brother, Ronnie, who gave of himself, outside of his occupation, without remuneration and without self-serving interests, and made life more enjoyable for young people.

Cartoons by Louis M. Conlin

Copyright © 1980
Clifford Bennett
All Rights Reserved

The Tiresias Press, Inc.
116 Pinehurst Ave., New York City 10033

International Standard Book Number: 0-913292-19-2
Library of Congress Catalog Card Number: 80-52650

Printed in U.S.A.

Current Printing (last digit) 10 9 8 7 6 5 4 3 2 1

Foreword

> "The aged are not a burden . . . . This is a home
> which is not just a place to eat and sleep but also a
> place where the aged can lead a life of their own."
> (Excerpt from a rest home brochure.)

The particular rest home described above closed its doors during
the mid-sixties, along with many others of its kind, to be replaced by an emerging nursing home industry that had the
financial base with which to comply and cope with rapidly
developing regulations for life safety, service expectations, and
spiraling costs of all kinds. "Homes" gave way to "long term
care facilities" with "levels of care," language indicating a shift
in physical design and service delivery modes. And with what
impact on the lives of those in need of those services and
facilities?

This book provides the necessary background with which to view the current state of institutional care for the elderly and to contrast that with what used to be and what should and could be. It is not, however, still another critique of the nursing home industry. It goes beyond that by offering the author's unique perspectives for looking at the elements of care in the nursing home setting and at how they affect residents' quality of life. These perspectives were gained from considerable personal and professional investments as both a nursing home patient and a nursing home administrator.

The humanism which permeates this work flows in part from Maslow's basic needs theory, the theoretical basis for the study which forms the core of the book. Validation of its application to nursing home life, and to the systems and dimensions of care which either support and nurture those needs or generate deficits in them, was pursued in both traditional and uniquely nontraditional study approaches. The uniqueness came from the author assuming the identity and thus the experiences of a nursing home patient, an approach necessary, in his view, to studying, analyzing, and proposing changes. The narration of these experiences, which the author relates to need satisfaction or deprivation, provides an exceptional texture to this book.

During a time when home care is enjoying a rebirth, Dr. Bennett risks taking the position that institutional care of the elderly can be refocused and guided to provide an environment which meets not only the most basic of human needs but those of a higher order which support the institutionalized older person in enjoying a quality of life which he so richly deserves. This book is about caring and respect for the elderly. It is about making nursing homes a *humanistic* alternative in elder care.

—Madeleine B. Provost, R.N., M.S.

Preface

This book was not written or motivated out of a desire to be critical of long term care facilities. Neither is it intended to defend or protect them. It is an objective analysis, presented from the perspective of one who has been both a nursing home administrator and a nursing home patient. How traditional homes came into being, the reasons why we have the kinds of long term care facilities that exist in our society today, and the myriad problems associated with them are dealt with. Appropriate solutions to improve care standards are included.

That there are deficiencies within the long term care system and injustices inflicted upon patients cannot be denied. Most administrators are honorable people who acknowledge that sad experiences sometimes happen to patients in their homes. The task of providing an environment which allows residents to have meaningful lives and good care, however, is a monumental one, for their medical and psychological needs are numerous, diverse, and complex. Homes do not deserve to be faulted for every unfortunate patient incident that occurs. It is the long term care system itself that bears responsibility for most of the failures and unfavorable episodes attributed to nursing homes. How and why this is so is dealt with in the pages that follow.

Of course, no health delivery system can entirely satisfy the physical and mental health requirements of all its patients. The aim of any health care component, therefore, is to satisfy the greatest number of people. Only when this is accomplished can the care service delivered be considered efficient and successful.

Quality of life is the primary concern of this book. In it, patients' needs are evaluated from *their* perspective and service delivery modes are presented which can help make the lives of older people more pleasant and worthwhile. Recommendations are made for changing established standards to improve patients' living environments.

Although all patients living in nursing homes would benefit greatly from the implementation of the ideas expressed in this book, there are some, particularly those suffering from senile dementia and other serious mental afflictions, who would benefit to a lesser degree. Their psychological state would deny them the opportunity to enjoy such basic human needs as total freedom and the power to make decisions. Their plight is unique and deserves intense research. The concepts presented are most meaningful when applied to the mentally alert patients who represent the majority of those in nursing homes.

The research and study forming the foundation for this book were done in skilled and intermediate care facilities created under federal guidelines. Although these institutions provide services for younger people, the current nursing home system was evolved for older people and it was for them that this book was written.

It is hoped that the ideas and concepts presented here will foster greater understanding of the many perplexing problems identified with nursing home life, and that this book will influence the long term care system to take a new direction and institute changes that will make a good quality of life for patients their highest priority.

—Clifford Bennett
Holyoke, Massachusetts, June, 1980

Acknowledgments

A book of this nature cannot be written without encouragement and assistance from many people. At the risk of overlooking someone, the following friends deserve special thanks:

Dr. Bertha Yanis Litsky, Consultant Microbiologist, to whom I will always be grateful for her years of friendship and interest in my career as a nursing home administrator.

Dr. Warren Litsky, Commonwealth Professor, University of Massachusetts, without whose inspiration, keen interest, and guidance it is doubtful that I would have started or completed this book.

Louis M. Conlin, Assistant Professor, Department of Education and Fine Arts, American International College. Professor Conlin's artistic talents are reflected in the cartoons in this book. I thank him for the many evening hours he spent converting my thoughts and ideas into quality illustrations.

Marcella Clark, Director of Nurses, Municipal Nursing Home of Holyoke, Massachusetts. I will always be thankful that Marcella was director of nurses for the nursing home where I gained most of my administrative experience. Her tolerance of me when I instituted changes in traditional operating routines contributed greatly to whatever success I may have had.

Barbara Morneau, Activities Director, Municipal Nursing Home of Holyoke, Massachusetts. Many of the concepts presented in this book were developed following the hours I spent with Barbara discussing the lives of nursing home patients. Her support, cooperation, interest, and encouragement are much appreciated.

Martin D. Moynihan, my eternal friend, who is known and respected for his aid to others. He was instrumental in my becoming a nursing home administrator.

My wife, Mary Claire, and my family. I will always feel guilty for having deprived them of my time during many days, weekends, holidays, and vacations while I carried out my professional responsibilities, studied, and wrote this book. I'm grateful, however, for their understanding, patience, and forgiveness.

Administration and faculty, Walden University, Naples, Florida. I am thankful for having had the opportunity to complete the advanced degree program at Walden. This university gave me the motivation I needed to study within my career field.

Patients and staffs of the nursing homes I administered. Because they were all so good to me, it is for them and for others like them that I have written this book.

Contents

PART I

1

Why the Need for Nursing Homes Will not Diminish

Nursing homes in the United States are often characterized by the media as deficient, misdirected, and in need of change. In an effort to stop injustices and to favorably influence the quality of patient care, television, newspapers, magazines, and books have alerted the public to abusive incidents occurring in long term care facilities. As a consequence, people think of nursing homes as bad and evil places. Fear of them has been ingrained in the minds of older people and of those who have relatives in need of that kind of service. Completion of life in one of them is represented as an unpleasant ending to productive and happy years.

This characterization, justified as it may sometimes be, alarms the public by emphasizing the negative aspects of long term care. Indeed, tragic circumstances and patient abuses do occur. They happen in every facility which provides 24-hour care for geriatric patients. But it is also true that tragedies occur in every part of our health system. The unnecessary operations, the unnecessary prescriptions, and the come-back schemes of some practicing physicians are well known. Understaffed hospitals are not rare, ambulances sometimes arrive too late, and medical laboratories sometimes fail to test specimens accurately.

Unfortunately, the reasons why substandard nursing homes exist, and *how* and *why* patients and their families have unpleasant experiences with them, are not being fully explained. Neither is the public being told of the difficult problems involved in delivering nursing home care, nor of the awesome responsibilities borne by nursing home personnel. As a result, misunderstandings have come about which adversely affect the reputations of many good and well-run facilities.

To understand how and why sad incidents happen in nursing homes, one must study the regulations that created them. Meaningful corrective alternatives can then be discussed. In its analysis of the nursing home system, this book attempts to demonstrate what the problems are and to offer suggestions to correct them.

The Rehabilitation Concept

It wasn't until the federal government passed Medicare and Medicaid legislation in 1965 that a positive effort was made to perfect care standards in nursing homes. Before this intervention, old and disabled persons were generally viewed as being unsalvable, although, of course, their medical disabilities were usually treated. Geriatrics, the treatment of physical diseases associated with old age, was (and still is) the accepted medical discipline applicable to the care of older patients.

Medicare and Medicaid brought forth care delivery requirements that extended the medical discipline of geriatrics to focus on rehabilitation. This came about because exponents of gerontological theories believed that many old people residing in nursing homes have restorative potential and that, through the use of various treatments and therapies, they can be returned to society. As a result, "rehabilitation" of the infirm aged has become fashionable. This is evidenced by regulations requiring elaborate physiotherapy departments in long term care facilities and by the employment of physical therapists and other rehabilitation specialists. It is also evidenced by the emergence of large, hospital-style geriatric institutions that proclaim their main responsibilities to be rehabilitation and treatment of disease.

Thus, currently, as in the past, the emphasis is on the physical-medical aspects of care for older people. Except for the requirement that homes have activities personnel to conduct diversionary recreational activity programs, little is being done to satisfy the many nonmedical needs of most patients. Nursing home systems, procedures, and environments are not changing or being modified to make the patients' lives more natural, livable, or meaningful. Built-in regulatory restraints, outdated medical modes, and inappropriate philosophies dominate the nursing home field and discourage long-overdue innovations.

Geriatrics, with its emphasis on medical care and restoration as the major objectives of nursing homes, is following a mistaken course. Most certainly there are some residents who can benefit from medical treatments and restorative therapies. Once the serious disabilities that are associated with old age strike, however, few are cured or rehabilitated. The great majority are not rehabilitatable. It is mainly those who have had recent disabling traumas who are able to return to their residences. Most all of the people admitted to homes reside there permanently, *never ever* to go home. It is this fact that everyone giving service to institutionalized older people should keep in mind. Since how patients live day to day is the real indicator of the quality of their care, disciplines that are nonmedical and socially oriented in nature should be given greater emphasis than those traditionally associated with geriatrics. These socially-oriented disciplines serve the greater number of residents. They are the main determinants of what good care is and what the important objectives of nursing homes should be.

The Community-Based Support Program Concept

Some health planners, principally individuals in federal and state government, believe that many older people confined to homes should not be there. They claim that the number of long term care beds should be reduced. The inference is that families commit relatives into homes unnecessarily and that community-based support programs can provide suitable care for older people outside of institutions. This is not true. Systems offering efficient community care have not been perfected. Families are deeply concerned and saddened by the experience of placing their loved ones in institutions. Most have sought every means

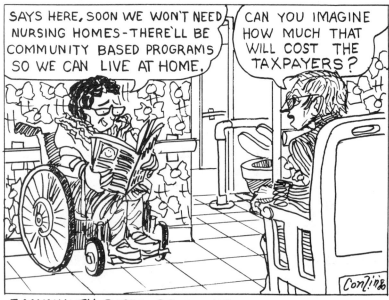

COMMUNITY BASED PROGRAMS.....

to avoid it, trying and exhausting all alternatives. It is typical that their mothers and fathers have been in and out of hospitals several times. Families admit their next of kin to nursing homes only as a last resort. In my 16 years as an administrator, I interviewed hundreds of family members of first-time patients and there were not more than two or three occasions when I suspected that alternate care could be provided in the community.

Those who believe that alternative measures should and can be employed to keep older disabled members of society living in their residences, view long term care facilities as an undesirable part of the health system and advocate letting them be phased out rather than making efforts to improve them. Support systems, such as homemaker services, home health aides, senior citizen centers, improved nutrition programs, improved transportation services, clinics, special housing, day care and night care centers, and other systems are offered as a means of accomplishing this goal. Thus, an illusion is being perpetrated which gives the impression that through the advent of these programs nursing homes will disappear for some magical reason and there is, therefore, little need to think about changing their designs and operating systems.

Why the Need for Nursing Homes Will not Diminish

Certainly, support programs have merit and can help many older people live longer in their communities. But the need for nursing homes is not going to diminish. Advancing medical science will extend more lives and the demand for nursing home beds will continue and, most likely, increase. Even if federal funding provides more systems and services to maintain older people in the community, many elders will still tire and accept institutionalization as the solution to their individual crises. Twenty-four-hour skilled medical care for large numbers of severely disabled old people who live in their own residences is not economically feasible. Also, it is reasonable to expect that the federal government will eventually take the position that the amount of money necessary to sponsor community-based programs, with their inevitable bureaucratic waste and inefficiency, makes nursing homes a sensible way to care for disabled elderly people. Not to be overlooked is the fact that nursing home care cost is considerably less than the cost of comprehensive community care. Ironically, the spending of federal money to develop alternatives to institutional care is delaying improvement of the lives of the many elderly people who now live in nursing homes.

2

The Changing Character
of the Nursing Home

A Look at the Past

Hundreds of years before Christ there were gathering places
where the sick, poor, aged, and indigent were cared for. It could
be said that these places were the remote ancestors of the
modern nursing home. During the Middle Ages, the Knights
Hospitalers (a monastic order from which the term "hospital"
is derived) played a significant role in expanding the number
of these institutions.

The beginnings of long term care facilities (nursing
homes) in America can be traced to the poorhouses, pest houses,
workhouses, and city and town infirmaries which were common in
the eighteenth and early nineteenth centuries. Some hospitals
that exist today were once forerunners of our current long term
care facilities. Pennsylvania Hospital in Philadelphia,
dating back to 1751, and Bellevue Hospital in New York City,
dating back to 1816, are examples. Both of these organizations

were founded to service the chronically ill, disabled, elderly, and diseased members of society.

These types of institutions existed well into the twentieth century. In 1908, for example, Massachusetts General Hospital stated that its purpose was to care for the sick, the aged, and the indigent. In fact, Holyoke's Massachusetts City and Town Infirmary, a facility I served, provided care for these kinds of people as late as the 1960s. Even at a later date some of the patients still thought of it as the poorhouse. I recall a woman patient saying to me, "I don't care what you say, Mr. Bennett, this is still the poorhouse."

The years between 1935 and 1955 were significant because it was in that period that actual nursing homes for the aged came into common use. Care for older people was more basic during this period and the health system was not as sophisticated as it is today. As in earlier days, many of the infirm elderly remained in hospitals when they had chronic disabilities and could not be cared for in their own homes. They were assigned to sections called "geriatric wards." But some, particularly those who were not acutely ill, were cared for in the nursing homes of the period, which were usually referred to as just plain "homes." They were not as numerous as homes are today and they differed considerably from those we have now. In fact, they possessed many desirable qualities not duplicated in modern facilities.

Typically, these homes were large, wooden residential structures. The bed capacities were small—20 or 30 beds were considered a lot. There was usually a large front porch and an attractive lawn or yard with shrubs and flowers. The owners and operators were ordinarily registered nurses who had seen an opportunity to fill a need and to earn income away from ordinary nursing duties. They were usually compassionate individuals who wanted to give disabled people more personal care than hospitals delivered.

These nurse-owned homes were less medically oriented than current geriatric institutions, and their environments were more social in style. Patients continued to be cared for under the direction of the family physician, who followed up with regular visits as needed. It was then an uncommon experience to have loved ones in a nursing home, and families maintained their close relationships with patients. Patients and family members were often seen sitting on the porches, passing the time, and watching the townsfolk going by. Eventually, however, strict construction standards and government-sponsored safety regulations made it almost impossible for this style of home to continue in business and there are relatively few of them operating today. Unfortunately, many of the good attributes and values of these facilities are now lost.

Actually, if we ask which came first, hospitals or nursing homes, we encounter a chicken-and-egg dilemma. Although the first hospitals were founded by benevolent citizens who wished to provide care for society's underpriviledged people, as medical science became more sophisticated hospitals deviated from this original purpose and abandoned the function of providing long term care for chronically ill and disabled people from nearby communities. This movement away from long term care for the sick coincided with a new dedication to the technical aspects of medical service, making the hospital "cure" oriented rather than "care" oriented. To fill the void created by this change in hospital philosophy, nursing homes increased in numbers and assumed responsibility for the care of the aged, disabled, and chronically ill. Ironically, if we compare the purpose for which nursing homes exist today with that of the earliest hospitals, it appears that the term "hospital" might be more appropriately applied to nursing homes and that today's hospitals should be called "special acute care facilities." As if to acknowledge this, many hospitals are now calling themselves "medical centers."

The Modern Nursing Home

It is significant that shortly after the advent of Medicare in 1965, hospitals gave an assist to the expansion of the nursing home industry outside of the established medical system. Demographic projections at the time predicted an increasing need for long term beds. Acute care facilities, which were expected to continue their long-standing interest in providing medical service to aged, disabled people, found themselves filled to capacity. Medical care costs were rising rapidly. To make beds available within the health system, and to hold care costs in line, the federal government encouraged existing medical facilities to build extended care facilities (ECFs). Under the Medicare program, the federal government would subsidize a major part of the cost of care for people over age 65 who were to use these new facilities. The patient day cost formulas for these ECFs were designed to establish daily rates which were less than prevailing hospital rates. The plan, therefore, was to reduce the overutilization of acute beds through the use of innovative hospital-based facilities for older people, and to reduce health costs by disallowing expenses associated with the more technical aspects of care.

Requirements for participation in this new program were strict, however, and expense elements, including construction costs, were controlled by the federal government. Hospitals preferred to remain independent and not get involved with the ECF system. Instead, they concentrated on increasing their emphasis on acute care. Consequently, the private sector—entrepreneurs, businessmen, and philanthropic organizations—filled the need. Nursing homes cropped up all over the country and a new segment of our health system was born. If the private sector had not taken advantage of this opportunity, long term care for thousands of elderly people would have been shamefully denied.

Levels of Care Classifications

In 1974, 23,000 facilities in the United States were classified as nursing homes. They provided beds for 1,235,000 patients. In 1985, there will be approximately 24,200 of these institutions with an estimated 1,296,800 patients. (This number does not include veterans' hospitals, state institutions, and other chronic care facilities which also serve geriatric cases). Public assistance programs, namely, Medicare and Medicaid, established special classifications for these institutions. The classifications are: Extended Care Facility (also called Intensive Nursing and Rehabilitative Care Facility)—Level I; Skilled Nursing Facility—Level II; Intermediate (or Supportive Nursing Care) Facility—Level III; and Resident Care (or Rest Home) Facility—Level IV. They differ basically by the amount of nursing personnel time required and the kinds and quantity of rehabilitation services, such as physiotherapy, occupational therapy, and specialized consultant services, that they deliver. The number of beds allowed per ward or section within a home also differs according to the classification. One or more levels of care may exist within a single nursing home. The level units or sections, however, must be distinct parts, separated from the others. Understanding these classifications will give some insight into many difficulties associated with nursing home care.

Classification Definitions

Level I. Extended Care Facility (Intensive Nursing and Rehabilitative Care Facility). Certified and approved for payment under Medicare. Serves those over age 65. The length of stay is limited under the Medicare guidelines. Cares for patients who have rehabilitation potential. Once it is determined by a utilization review committee that a patient will not benefit from rehabilitation services, she or he must be transferred to a Level

III facility.

Must be under the direction of a licensed nursing home administrator and have a licensed physician medical director. Twenty-four hour supervision under the direction of a professional registered nurse is required. The services of a social worker, audiologist, speech therapist, and physiotherapist must be available. Various consultant services, such as those provided by a dietician and a pharmacist, must be available. A physician must visit each patient at least once every 30 days.

Patients assigned to this level must require medical care that is considered skilled. Examples of such services are: intravenous injections, intravenous feedings, and insertion and replacement of indwelling catheters. These facilities may have dialysis machines.

Level II. Skilled Nursing Care Facility. May or may not be certified under Medicare. If not, payments will not be covered by Medicare. This nursing home is approved for payments under public assistance programs such as Medicaid. Patients must have rehabilitation potential or require skilled care to remain in this level. As in the case of Level I, a utilization review committee may transfer patients to Level III.

Standards are the same as those for Level I.

Level III. Intermediate Care Facility (or Supportive Nursing Care Facility). Not certified under Medicare. Payments are, however, provided under Medicaid. The utilization review committee may determine that the services are not needed for a patient and require his or her transfer to a Level IV facility or back to the community.

The degree of medical service needed by patients is less than that available in Skilled Nursing Care Facilities. Patients require 24-hour supervision or observation and need services of nursing personnel. Examples of intermediate care are: recording vital signs, administering dressings, and dispensing oral medications. The facility must be under the direction of a professional registered nurse and have a consultant licensed physician. Other limited consultant services are required. A physician must visit each patient once every 90 days.

Level IV. Resident Care Facility (Rest Home). Provides for payments under the Supplementary Social Security Program (SSI). The facility gives room and board and very limited nursing services.

How Patients Are Assigned to Levels of Care

Sixty percent (13,700) of nursing homes in the United States are in the skilled and intermediate categories (Levels I, II, and III), with 9,245 being skilled and 4,455 being intermediate. This book deals mainly with these two kinds of facilities. It was in skilled nursing homes with intermediate care components that I gained experience and did research, and it is on these facilities that attention is being focused here. The concepts presented, however, apply to all classifications because they all have one thing in common: they all provide care and service to older human beings. Regardless of the level to which people are assigned, they all need to enjoy a peaceful and meaningful life. Patients' needs can be satisfied or deprived in any institution.

When patients are assigned to particular levels of care, they are required to reside in those levels. In other words, it is irregular to assign patients to Level III and have them live in Level II.

The Utilization Review Process

The classification of patients by level of care, and their assignments to corresponding beds, involves a very complex process. The initial classifications start with the attending physicians, whose diagnoses and prognoses establish the extent of care or treatments needed and, hence, what the patients' levels will be. Physicians can manipulate or swing the diagnoses and prognoses and consciously earmark patients for desired classifications. Bed availability, the physicians' personal and professional appraisal of the circumstances involved, and family considerations can influence their evaluations. They can, and sometimes do, maneuver patients' medical needs to qualify them for admittance to favored nursing homes.

All facilities certified under Medicare and Medicaid employ a utilization review (UR) system. Hospitals, for example, have UR committees (which include nurse specialists) that monitor physician-assigned classifications. The purpose is not only to check the doctors' assessments of the cases but, most particularly, to hasten discharges whenever possible and transfer patients to nursing homes. This often creates conflicts between the physicians, who may sincerely believe that some patients should remain in the hospital, and the UR committees, who believe they should leave. Physicians may be under pressure to hold their clients in the hospital until families arrange suitable accommodations in the community or in a desired nursing home. Hospitals' cost containment efforts place pressure on UR committees to reduce the utilization of beds. Here again, the diagnoses and prognoses and resultant classification levels can be swung, either by the physicians or by UR personnel, to either keep patients in the hospital or effect a transfer to homes happening to have vacancies in certain levels.

Once a patient is transfered to a nursing home, the UR process goes on. Homes conduct case reviews (reviews of patients' medical and social histories) in conjunction with UR committees. Level I and II cases are reviewed every 30 days. Level III cases are reviewed every 90 days. There is a dual purpose for this: first, to monitor patients' care plans and prescribed treatments; and second, to verify that the patients' level classifications are correct. Conflicts grow between the attending physicians and the facilities over these case reviews. Volumes and volumes of paperwork are accumulated to carry out these procedures. Patients, their families, and their physicians undergo a variety of disheartening experiences. When it is determined that certain medical characteristics of patients have changed, the patients are moved from level to level and from place to place. All this results in harassment for everyone involved, and in waste and a juggling of papers to perpetuate a system that doesn't work. Hospitals may need a mechanism to avoid unnecessary utilization of their beds, but using URs for the purpose of determining if nursing home patients have the correct bed assignments is frivolous and unessential. Most patients will never, ever leave the nursing home. What home, or what particular section of a home they live in is unimportant. They need quality care and service wherever they reside. The attending physician alone can, after consultation with a patient and his or her family, decide whether nursing home care is needed. If it is, the home should be chosen on the basis of the quality of service it delivers rather than on impersonal level classifications.

Types of Ownership

Nursing homes also differ on the basis of ownership. The two basic kinds of ownership are private and nonprofit. Private homes may be syndicated (which means that a corporation owns many homes) or individually owned. The individually-owned facility may be an incorporated institution or a proprietorship. The nonprofit organizations fall into two categories—those sponsored by government and those sponsored by private corporations. The figure on the next page illustrates the system of homes in the United States. Seventy-seven percent of the homes in this country are privately owned. The balance of 23 percent are sponsored by nonprofit religious, governmental, or philanthropic organizations.

The type of ownership is not evidence of quality of care. There are excellent and substandard homes in every category. A good home is the product of the work of the staff, principally the professional registered nurses, licensed practical nurses, nurses' aides and others. They determine if the needs of the patients are satisfied to the highest degree possible. Most importantly, they are the people who distribute compassion, empathy, and concern among the patients and their families. And it is they who must struggle to overcome the many limitations and restraints placed upon homes by the system itself. Consciencious and caring employees are found in every type of nursing facility.

Nonprofit homes are frequently thought to give superior care and to have lower per diem rates than others. The assumption is that the monies they earn or the donations made to them go back to the patients in the form of services and that, therefore, no profit it made. This is one of the many false assumptions made about the nursing home system. No home is operated to generate a loss. Both kinds of organizations, profit and nonprofit, are administered to maximize their incomes. The goals are the same—to deliver quality service in the most cost-efficient way. All homes try to minimize expenses and maximize the patients' daily rates. The operating standards controlling personnel staffing patterns, support systems, and physical environments provide the framework for optimum care. The federal guidelines are the same for all nursing homes. There is simply no logical reason why one type of home should deliver better services than another when they all operate under the same regulations and standards. Homes that receive adverse publicity because of their poor care standards are those that are

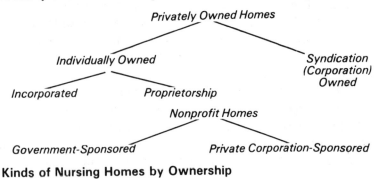

Kinds of Nursing Homes by Ownership

not effectively monitored by state health agencies to make certain that the prevailing guidelines are adhered to.

All nursing homes suffer a "philosophical conflict" between the effort to deliver optimum care and the effort to reduce operating costs. If this conflict is stated in the form of a question—how can enough money be spent to meet the needs of all the patients while, at the same time, care costs are kept to a minimum?—it is obvious that it can't be resolved.The needs of patients are too numerous and cost containment controls are too strict to permit the delivery of ideal service.

The outstanding difference between profit and nonprofit organizations is how this philosophical conflict is resolved; specifically, how the profits are used. In the case of private homes, they go to the proprietors or stockholders. Nonprofit facilities place the excess income in reserve accounts, investments, and sometimes into cost elements, such as salaries for key personnel, special equipment, or maintenance of the buildings. There are advantages and disadvantages to each of these profit distribution options. Private homes generally have lower per diem rates, lower operating costs, and conservative financial controls. Not-for-profit homes generally have higher rates and higher operating costs but enjoy a reputation of giving excellent care. The merits of each of these systems and the quality of the services delivered by them are subjects for individual interpretations and endless debates.

The Need for Change
Advances in medicine and changes within the family structure have had profound effects on our older population, effects which demonstrate the need to consider changes within the nursing home system. Vital statistics of the U.S. Department of Health, Education, and Welfare indicate that the average life expectancy is now 79.3 years, whereas in 1900 it was only 46.3 years. More people live to old age than ever before. Ten percent

of our population (20 million persons) are now 65 or older. With new medical discoveries and improved health care, it is expected that 25 percent of the population will be candidates for institutional services in the year 2000.

One who is admitted to a nursing home can expect to live there for about two years—the average length of stay before death comes. Many will spend three, five, ten, or more years in residence. It is reasonable to expect that these lengths of stay will increase in the future.

After their children are grown, people live independent lives for more years than in earlier times. The economic needs of their sons and daughters—the need for both wife and husband to work in order to own a home and a car or two and to educate their children—make it difficult for them to take care of their parents during their final years. No longer is it the custom for the oldest daughter to remain unmarried and be the nurse-housekeeper until death arrives at the household to set her free. Thus, the nursing home is, and will remain, the catchment basin for the elderly who, for a variety of reasons, cannot satisfy their care needs in the community.

Other significant events have taken place in society which will contribute to a continuing demand for nursing home beds. The Social Security laws of 1965 greatly affect this need. As long as federal money (Medicare or Medicaid) is used to support nursing homes, anyone, regardless of his or her financial resources, may seek admittance to any home in the country regardless of where he or she may live. No home, unless it has no beds for the applicant's classification level, has the legal basis to refuse a person who qualifies under government programs. The stigma of placing loved ones in a nursing home has been removed—it is now socially acceptable. Reliance on these facilities for the care of Mother and Father during their final years is *an experience facing every American family.* The appropriateness of nursing home patients' lifestyles and the operating standards and environments of these institutions should be the concern of every American citizen.

Nursing homes in the United States, regardless of their organizational structure, still face many of the problems that their predecessors, the poorhouses, did a hundred years ago. They are still places where old and infirm persons are placed and where sick people go when they cannot afford medical or supportive care in the community.

It may be argued that this is not true, that nursing homes are far better than the old poorhouses because they are better constructed and because medical care is more advanced than it used to be. Granting that this is so, still, if we compare the quality of life of today's institutionalized older people with their lifestyles before admittance, and if we consider today's great resources, it is evident that serious deficiencies related to their care still exist. As in the past, there is much more that can be done for them. The questions currently facing society are: are nursing home patients' needs being satisfied to the fullest extent, and are they living in the kind of environments they deserve? It is my contention that they are still very much deprived and that their living conditions should be improved. Homes may be better constructed, and medical science may have advanced, but research on improving the quality of life for nursing home patients is still neglected. Regulatory restraints have forced homes to have static environments. Relative disinterest is being shown by federal and state health agencies toward many of the environmental conditions associated with long term care facilities. Consequently, the negative image of nursing homes will remain until new standards are implemented to make improving the patients' quality of life the major concern of governmental health officials and the nursing home industry.

Systems and procedures need to be reevaluated and changed to satisfy a multitude of unmet patients' needs. At the same time, costs having no direct bearing on the quality of care (the levels of care system, for example) should be eliminated. Regulated conservatism is misdirecting the nursing home system and perpetuating practices that have been in vogue for all too many years. One needs only to look at the kinds of facilities being built today to be made aware of this. There hasn't been a basic interior style change since Medicare was legislated. Construction standards have been principally the same since 1965, except for added restraints such as the life safety code requirements, which increase construction costs and inhibit conceptual innovation.

Admittedly, homes are constructed better today than ever before and there are many well-built and visually attractive buildings. But good construction materials, safety devices, and colorful decors do not mean that the occupants are being given a livable environment. It is the interior configuration of the bricks and mortar, the space allotments, the internal designs, and the personnel procedures that are the real indicators of a good home. To understand why this is so, traditional home environments and the kind of lives patients have living in them must be studied. Analyses of this kind will determine if the system sponsors appropriate care and if it is preparing for the hundreds of thousands of older people who will live and die in nursing homes in coming years.

How patients live in today's homes should be part of society's consciousness. Old people must not be made to live an existence that is not worthwhile. They have spent too many years as viable tax-paying members of society and have made too many contributions toward our way of life to end under wretched circumstances. Institutionalization should not represent a loss of their rights to be free and productive to their maximum potential. Neither should it be an end, but rather a new period where they can live out their final years in peace and have the opportunity to satisfy their individual needs as they once did.

As one who has been part of the long term care system for many years, I submit that traditional nursing homes, including the homes I administered, fail to meet the basic human needs of patients. Inappropriately designed, employing inappropriate systems and procedures, they were created mainly to provide expedient measures for the care of disabled older people. This expedience on the part of the nursing home system has sacrificed the human values of the human beings they serve. Responsibility for this rests with misguided architects and health planners, particularly individuals in federal and state governments, who influenced existing nursing home regulations. They failed to do the necessary research to ensure that construction standards and care procedures would respect patients' basic human needs.

That the environments of homes have not been of primary concern to planners is exemplified by the fact that these facilities emulate hospitals. Life in a medically-oriented, acute care setting has been deemed adequate for nursing home residents. Whether or not such an environment is conducive to the satisfaction of patients' basic human needs has not been questioned. The residents of homes are expected to abandon their prior lifestyles, their possessions, and their independence to live in "homes" that, with their long corridors, small rooms, and employment of acute care medical procedures, resemble hospitals. This is indeed a cruel development and one of the many concerns that provoked me to write this book. Subsequent chapters will elaborate on specific aspects of the traditional environments, the resulting deprivations of patients, and methods to improve the delivery of care in nursing homes.

3

Basic Human Needs of Residents

The preceding chapters have made some references to *basic human needs* and *quality of life*. Actually, they are rather unclear terms, subject to many interpretations.

Identifying and defining these terms became important to me several years ago. I had seen them in the medical literature but wasn't quite sure how they related to the people living in the facility I administered. It seemed that, in order to determine if my staff was using appropriate service delivery modes and if the environment of the home was conducive to a good life for the patients, a clear understanding of these terms was vital. I hypothesized that *when patients' basic human needs are satisfied, they enjoy a good quality of life.* To examine this hypothesis, I carried out the following effort.

How Basic Human Needs Were Studied
The first task was to identify and isolate the patients' basic human needs. I believed these had to be made specific so that

anyone working in the home would know precisely what they were. Abraham H. Maslow's heirarchy of needs theory was used as a starting point for the study. Maslow's concept is widely accepted by the social science and management fields and has been adopted by many in the health sciences. Never before, however, has it been equated with the total nursing home environment in a cause and effect relationship to determine if the facility enhances or inhibits patients' satisfaction of their needs.

This concept is presented in pyramid form and graphically shows five levels of human needs. It theorizes that man satisfies his needs in order of priority and that one must successfully achieve the first level of needs before seeking to satisfy the second-level needs. As the lower needs are gratified, one progresses to the higher levels, by order of priority, until self-actualization is finally attained. By correlating the nursing home environment with Maslow's pyramid, it is evident that long term

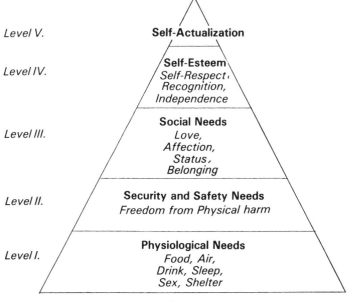

Maslow's Heirarchy of Needs

care facilities are designed and operated to satisfy first- and second-level (physiological; security and safety) needs. But what of the higher needs?

Assisting me with the study were three members of my staff at the 134-bed Municipal Nursing Home of Holyoke in Massachusetts. They were the director of nurses, the activities director, and the social worker. They were experienced people, with an average of 11 years of working with nursing home patients. Each of them had exhibited an abundance of compassion and concern for the patients. They were dedicated and loyal people who were highly motivated to improve the nursing home environment.

After a great deal of deliberation, it became evident that Maslow's theory did not precisely identify our patients' basic needs. It was too ambiguous for our purpose and did not relate

		List of Assumed Basic Human Needs Correlated with Maslow's Pyramid Levels
Self-Actualization	*Level V.*	Accomplishment
Self-Esteem Independence, Recognition, Self-Respect	*Level IV.*	Freedom, Privacy, Independence, Decision-Making, Choice of food, Choice of clothes, Recognition, Control over financial affairs
Social Needs Love, Belonging, Affection, Status	*Level III.*	Family, Friends, Religion, Possessions, Communication, Community involvement, Purchasing
The items below were dropped from the study.		
Safety and Security Needs Freedom from Physical Harm	*Level II.*	Freedom from physical harm
Physiological Needs Food, Air, *Drink*, Sleep, Sex, Shelter	*Level I.*	Meals, Drinks, Sleep, Sex, Air, Warmth, Medicine, Medicine, Medical Services

specifically to long term care patients. The only way to clarify the dilemma was to ask the patients themselves how they perceived their needs. To accomplish this, a list of *assumed needs,* which could be correlated with Maslow's theory but which were more specific to the nursing home environment, was developed. These were then positioned opposite the corresponding levels of the pyramid to justify their use as attainment goals. The needs identifiable with the physiological and the safety and security levels at the base of the pyramid were dropped from the study because traditional nursing homes are administered to satisfy them. Sex and love were dropped from the study because of their complexity. It was felt that they merited independent investigation and analysis. The list devised for the research effort, along with clarifying definitions, is as follows:

Assumed Needs and Clarifying Definitions

accomplishment—(to achieve something)
freedom—(to move about and do things)
privacy—(having the option of being alone)
independence—(doing things for oneself)
making decisions—(deciding for oneself what one wants)
recognition—(others' interest in one)
control over own financial affairs—(knowledge of, and a say in, one's own financial affairs)
family—(seeing one's family)
friends—(seeing one's friends)
religion—(participating in one's religion)
communication with people outside the nursing home—(freedom to contact people outside the home)
possessions—(having one's own belongings with one)
community activities—(being involved with community life)
shopping and buying—(being able to buy things)
choice of what to wear—(having enough clothes available from which to choose what one will wear)
choice of food—(being able to have a say about what one eats)

The Need Selection Process

After establishing the list of assumed needs, the next effort was to obtain patients' responses to them. First, however, it had to be determined which patients would be included in the study. Because many had afflictions which limited their ability to respond, the number of participants had to be controlled. Patients with severe speech impediments, severe hearing loss, poor eyesight, acute illness, and distinct emotional and mental handicaps were declared nonparticipatory. The most able and alert people were wanted so that there would be no question of their ability to understand what the questions were and why we were asking them.

To decide which patients would take part, a list of all 134 patients living in the facility was reviewed by the special committee. Twenty-five people were selected who were believed to be mentally alert and physically and emotionally able to respond. They were then queried individually by me in a private room.

Each of the 16 assumed patient needs, along with the short clarifying statements, were printed in large, black letters on two by-six-inch yellow cards.   They were placed in random order on table in front of each interviewee. The resident was then asked, "Do you agree or disagree that some, or all, of the cards represent things that are important to you and are basic human needs of nursing home patients?" All 25 patients stated that they were, indeed, basic human needs of nursing home patients. We had now established a usable list of needs for research into the lives of elderly people living in long term care institutions.

Establishing a Priority of Needs

The next task was to establish an order of priority for the needs. This would indicate which ones the patients thought were most important and should receive particular attention. To accomplish this, each patient interviewee was asked to arrange the cards in order of importance. The findings were then tallied.

The priority of needs, as determined by the patients, was:

possessions
family
freedom
privacy
independence
making decisions
choice of food
friends
choice of what to wear
religion
control over own financial affairs
communication with people outside the home
recognition
community activities
shopping and buying
accomplishment

The results of this experiment were most revealing. That possessions would be considered number one in priority and accomplishment last was a surprise. In any event, a list of components had been obtained that could be evaluated and equated with the nursing home environment to determine if patients' basic human needs were being satisfied. These needs are discussed at length in Chapter 7.

Information gained from the study was immediately transmitted to the entire staff of the facility. The data became part of the frequent training programs conducted for employees in every department. For the first time, objectives could be discussed in positive terms.

Since plans for renovating the existing building and constructing a new 120-bed facility were in the formative stages, the staff became enthusiastic about having an opportunity to influence the construction of an innovative home that would be specially designed to satisfy patients' needs as defined by the research. But their innovative suggestions encountered frustrating resistance. For example, it became clear that the common practice of squeezing in the maximum number of beds into a facility would take precedence over the patients' needs for privacy. In addition, the need for patients to have bureaus in their rooms for possessions and surface space on which they could place mementos and family photographs could not be satisfied because the rooms, as recommended by the developers, were not large enough. Surprisingly, the requirement for this essential piece of furniture had been waived by the Massachusetts Department of Public Health and dropped completely from the renovation and construction plans. As has been the case historically, the patients' needs and their lifestyles were of secondary importance. There were many progressive things that could have been done, but suggested changes that deviated from traditional ways were faced with the customary lack of knowledge about nursing home patients and with antiquated ideas. It became evident that the new facility would *not* be innovative and would be designed according to the traditional medical model.

Despite this setback, I continued to be involved in lengthy discussions with my activities director and director of nurses over strategies to effect changes which would improve the quality of life of institutionalized older people. During one of these conferences, my activities director suddenly said to me, "You know, only patients truly understand the lives of patients. Why don't you admit yourself into a nursing home and become a patient?" I was shocked, but it seemed like one hell of a good idea. At that moment, she started a train of events that would have profound effects on my thinking. Ultimately, a scheme was developed for me to enter a home incognito where I would experience the real life of a nursing home patient. This highly emotional and enlightening experience is covered in detail in Part II, which follows.

PART II
4

The Author's Experience as a Nursing Home Resident

Reflections Before the Admittance

For several months I carried in my mind the idea of becoming a nursing home patient. At times it seemed unreal and not something that could come about. Sometimes I thought an experience of this kind was unnecessary because it would probably only confirm what I already knew. Of course, I had preconceived ideas about patients' needs; after all, I had been concerned about them for many years. Like most administrators, I believed I ran a good home and was genuinely concerned about patients and their needs. So perhaps going into a home might only be an exercise in justifying my opinions. Besides, I questioned my nerve and the wisdom of subjecting myself to such an experiment. As part of the process of resolving my conflicting feelings about the project, I reflected upon my professional responsibilities during the previous years.

The responsibilities of managing a nursing home are very diverse. Unlike hospitals, which have large and sophisticated administrative support staffs, a home depends largely on the expertise of the administrator. He has to be intimately involved with, and knowledgeable about, every department. Very often, as in my case, he has no assistant and every department reports directly to him. He has to be familiar with the business activities of the general office and totally knowledgeable about federal and state regulations and all operating policies. In addition, he has to understand the sanitary procedures used by the housekeeping staff, oversee the purchasing of all the supplies, and comprehend the psychological and sociological concepts employed in the nursing, social service, and activities departments. In particular, he has to be a skilled supervisor who is familiar with and uses all of the latest supervisory and management techniques.

The home I administered was a good facility and enjoyed an excellent reputation among people living in the community. Even though it was publicly owned, it had operated within its income for the past six years—an unusual accomplishment. Under my administration, enough surplus capital was generated so that plans could be formulated to renovate the building and construct what was supposed to be the most up-to-date facility in the country.

I and my entire staff were concerned with the environment and the day-to-day living conditions of the patients. Together we explored ways to make life better for them. We conducted surveys and educational programs, and experimented with innovative service delivery modes. Most of the time we accomplished our goals.

It frequently occurred to me that I should be less involved with the patients and their families. Being satisfied with traditional ways and occupying myself with economic and material factors would be less demanding. Simply applying my time to managing the routine problems of running the nursing home would be an easier course to follow.

Yet, as time passed, I came to realize that my activities director's suggestion was a good one because there was a part of the patients' lives I could not grasp. A real understanding of what it was like to be a patient was missing and the only way to gain that understanding, obviously, was to become a patient myself. Then I would learn firsthand what a resident's day-to-day life is like and could, from a patient's point of view, monitor the effectiveness of the operating systems and procedures used to satisfy patients' needs, learn why tragic incidents happen to patients and how measures can be adopted to prevent them, and find out how nursing home systems and environments deprive elderly people. I would then be in a position to return to my facility with fresh ideas and more realistic perspectives, ready to institute needed changes.

The Plan

With the decision finally made, I was burdened with logistical problems. The more I considered the experiment, the more complicated it became. I had thought that the most difficult part would be finding a nursing home into which I could be admitted. I had lectured in various parts of the region and this presented the possibility of my being recognized during my stay in a home. The home, therefore, would have to be far removed from where I was best known.

I would need the assistance of an innovative and fearless administrator—the kind of person who could understand that my intentions were constructive and that collecting bad tales was the last thing on my mind because I had a ready supply of them at my own facility. In time, I spoke to an outstanding administrator who ran a large nursing home in a distant part of the region. When I explained my plan to him, he responded enthusiastically, "Great! You can use my home and I'll help you."

Now the scheme was finally becoming a reality. It was also becoming somewhat frightening and I was beginning to feel apprehensive and reluctant. The thought of changing my identity was causing me anxiety because I had never acted before or pretended to be someone else.

With the home selection out of the way, the final details had to be planned. The idea that originally seemed simple became complex. There were so many things to think about and anticipate. It became evident that I could not handle the planning alone. I had to solicit support, advice, and assistance from some understanding friends.

Although they helped me with the planning, these people were divided as to whether or not I should follow through with the experiment. One of them was worried about the psychological impact it would have on me. Another tried to impress on me the potential hazards involved and frequently said, "It's going to be a lot harder than you think." A third was very concerned and expressed her feelings by saying, "I don't think you should do it, but if you do, make sure you know what you are doing." A fourth was reserved. He counselled me on the consequences but wanted me to make up my own mind. He thought, however, that a real contribution could be made to nursing homes by such an investigation. The fifth, an attorney, was enthusiastic and offered his support. My wife, Mary, was reassuring as she always is, and simply let me do what I wanted to do, even though I would be using my annual vacation time away from her and our family. Although my advisors had conflicting ideas, they gave me support and helped to complete the details of the admittance plan.

Many factors had to be taken into consideration. One was the length of time to be spent in the home. How much exposure would I need to view the total nursing home environment? It was decided that ten days would be appropriate. This would take me through a weekend, and I would gain experience both during peak activity hours and slower periods. Other factors to be considered were: creating a new identity along with a family history; developing a medical history which would qualify me as a nursing home patient; planning how to cut off any effort by personnel at the facility to research my background and thereby expose my identity; and finding a method to get me in and out of the home incognito. After many hours of planning, the following procedure was devised:

1. The medical diagnosis would be that of an alcoholic with a history of stomach trouble, asthma, and edema in the left leg (I had a little edema).
2. The first few days would be spent in a wheelchair with the left leg extended.
3. I would go unshaven for a few days, wear old clothes, use my old pair of glasses, discard my dentures, and give the appearance of a typical alcoholic.
4. The admittance would be to a Level II bed.
5. I would be admitted under an assumed name.
6. My family would not be involved.
7. The admittance would be considered a referral from an agency.
8. A friend, carrying the physician's referral and medical forms, would drive me to the nursing home.
9. The admittance papers would indicate that my friend had located another home to which I would be transferred in ten days.
10. The director of nursing and the business manager of the facility would be alerted to the scheme to prevent internal research on my physical history.
11. All parties involved would pledge confidentiality and secrecy.
12. The experiment would be instantaneously aborted if the secret became known.
13. My notes about the nursing home environment, the patients, my experience, and the operational systems would be mailed to a friend every day.

Early one spring day, with a two-day's growth of beard, dressed in old clothes, wearing an old pair of glasses, and with an old suitcase by my side, I phoned the administrator of the home where I was to stay and said to him, "Here I come." He answered heartily, "Come on!" I then set out by car, with my friend at the wheel, to spend what turned out to be ten intensely emotional but revealing days in a nursing home.

The Admittance Experience

The leisurely automobile ride to the nursing home was overshadowed by feelings of apprehension. My friend asked me on several occasions, "Are you sure you want to do this?" Although I replied in the affirmative, I really wanted to turn around. For one thing, I was still worried that someone would recognize me at the facility I was going to. I had no feeling of being disguised even though I had a heavy beard and was wearing shabby clothes.

As the car proceeded, I reflected on the significance of such a trip to the thousands of people who have had this experience. Their nursing home stays involved no time frame and probably had a fearful termination. It seemed logical that older folks, while being taken to a nursing home for residency, must have mental flashbacks and think about their past histories. *I* thought about my work, my family, and the consequences of sacrificing ten days of my vacation time. Certainly, *they* must think of the years when they were younger and how long life seemed when they were children. Their whole life, I imagined, must come before their eyes—their parents, upbringing, educational pursuits, occupational endeavors, children, successes, and failures. Could anything have prepared them for the events about to befall them?

The engine had hardly stopped when a wheelchair was brought to the car and my door was opened. A nurse reached in, touched my arm, and said, "I'll help you get into the chair." In seconds, I was being pushed through the opened front entryway. I had become a nursing home patient. I thought, "I'm going in for ten days—how must it be for those who know they are going in for the rest of their lives?'' Experience told me that most do, indeed, know this.

I was wheeled into the admittance office, a small room with one desk for the admitting nurse. The nurse, seated in her swivel chair, was handed my medical history and other supporting papers. She was extremely kind and concerned. I'd been admitted to hospitals, but this was different. Hospital atmospheres are sterile and the personnel can be quite businesslike, impersonal, and cold. This nurse's voice reflected compassion and understanding for my predicament. She assured me that I would be all right and that everyone working in the facility would do

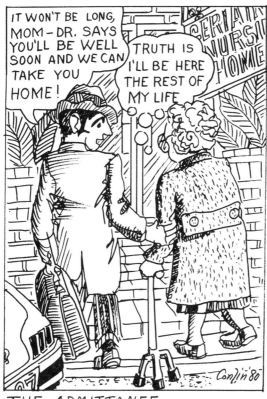

THE ADMITTANCE....

their best to take care of me. She even asked me about my eating habits, and told me I could have coffee or tea any time I wished. If I had any unusual problems, I was simply to make them known to the staff and they would respond. To test her, I asked for a glass of beer. She was a little startled and, obviously, had to turn down my request. Then I compromised and asked for a cup of tea. A phone call was immediately made to the dietary department and in a few minutes a kitchen worker came into the room and handed me a hot cup of tea. It was clear that the admitting nurse was trying her best to make me feel secure in my new surroundings. As assuring as she was, however, I was getting nervous in anticipation of what was yet to come. When my friend left to start on the long drive back home, for some unexplainable reason I almost cried. It was as though it was *really* happening!

The admitting nurse wheeled me out of her office to take me to my bedroom. She told me that I would be sharing it with a patient named Mr. Johnson, a victim of Parkinson's disease. She pushed me through the lobby, down a corridor, and around two corners to an elevator, introducing me on the way to several staff members, each of whom made a reassuring comment.

When the elevator stopped at the desired floor, I was wheeled around a corner and down a corridor to a nursing station, where I was introduced to several nurses and aides. Then I was taken to a two-bed room where I was introduced to 75-year-old Mr. Johnson. By this time I had lost all sense of direction and had no idea in which part of the facility I was—it was as though I had been taken to my room blindfolded.

This introduction to the nursing home environment was the start of many days of periodic confusion and disorientation. My anxieties and deep concerns over what I was doing and my frustration over what I was learning interferred with my ability to cope with the experience in a purely rational way. Now I knew what it was like to be committed to a nursing home.

The usual admittance procedure continued. My clothes

were checked by two nurses, who, after noting each article on a piece of paper, placed the article in a bureau drawer. Personal items were taken from my dilapidated suitcase and neatly put in my bedside stand. I was then instructed on how to use the nurse call bell. It was made clear that I must use the bell and not attempt to get out of the wheelchair alone. The nurses did not want to risk a fall by an unstable and shaking patient.

The next phase of the procedure was to orient me to my surroundings. This is standard procedure when a patient is admitted to an institution. I was introduced to the lavatory, the clothes closet, the call bell a second time, the sink, and the over-the-bed table. It was essential that I be made aware of all the equipment that I would be using. Then I was wheeled out of the bedroom, past the nursing station, down the corridor, around a corner, and into an attractively decorated lounge where a television set was playing.

Most of the patients in the lounge were in wheelchairs. Some had walkers, and a few were slouched in upholstered chairs. I felt disturbed and out of place and I started to question my staying power for the next nine days. Not having a watch, I had lost track of the time and had to ask my escort nurse what it was. Then, after introducing me to several of the more alert patients, she left.

Only two hours had passed since I had entered the facility. I had come to a place that many old people are told is to be their home. But I did not feel I was in a "home." Clearly, it was a medical facility, more like a hospital—a place where one comes, not to live, but to die!

Analyzing a Nursing Home—the First Day

The moment had come for me to reflect on the experience and prepare for notetaking as planned. All of the important variables of the study came to mind—my feelings, the attitudes of the patients and staff, how I and the staff related to the environment, and how the patients' basic human needs were met. Until then, I had not fully realized how multidimensional my experiment would be. The task was more complex than I had anticipated. I would have to be an analyst, a patient, and an imposter all at the same time.

To my consternation, an element had been overlooked in developing the admittance plan. I had worn an old pair of glasses so I would experience what nursing home life is like to an older person with unsuitable lenses. In addition, I had to keep my hands shaking to prove to the staff that I was an alcoholic. Under these conditions, how could notes be taken? I realized that I would have to do my notetaking privately.

It was during my initial stay in the lounge that I became friendly with Mr. Gray, another patient. He became interested in me immediately, wanting to know where I came from, where I had worked, if I was married and had children, and how I got there. I told him I hadn't worked for years, had no family, was an alcoholic, and had been sent into the home by an agency. He insisted that I was too young to be in a nursing home and urged me to get better quickly and get out, get a job, get married, and raise a family. This conversation, one of many in which I was forced to be untruthful, provoked severe guilt feelings.

Mr. Gray was about 65 years old, in relatively good physical condition, and fully ambulatory. For the last few years he had been depressed and suicidal. He related to me, detail by detail, how he had attempted suicide twice, the last time by jumping off the roof of a four-story building. Miraculously, he had only broken some bones, which were now almost mended. Yet, troubled and sad as he was, he was concerned about my welfare. Having had some experience with suicidal persons, I questioned whether he was getting the type of care he needed. Since he had tried suicide twice, I knew that without the proper help he might succeed the third time. Nursing home professionals are not usually trained or experienced to handle Mr. Gray's kind of problem—psychiatric services are not normally part of nursing home care. I thought it a real imposition on the nursing staff for him to be there since, should he harm himself, they would be held accountable. It was also unfair to him, for he should have had a more specialized type of care.

After I had been in the lounge for almost an hour, the supper carts started arriving in the ward. A nurses' aide pushed me back to my bedroom where I was to await the arrival of my supper tray. Then I had my first encounter with inappropriate nursing home architecture. I had to use the lavatory to which I had been introduced earlier that afternoon. Remembering the order to use the call bell, I rolled myself along the side of my bed to reach for it. That proved to be very difficult because the over-the-bed table was in my way. One has to try to maneuver an over-the-bed table while seated in a wheelchair to appreciate the complications involved. It is no wonder, I thought, that some patients who try to do this tumble head first out of their wheelchairs—and then get tied in them for protective reasons! I did at last manage to reach the bell and in a few minutes an aide arrived in my room.

Upon request, the aide pushed me to the lavatory door. It opened out, as many toilet doors do in nursing homes, and only after several attempts and some banging of the door and its frame, did she manage to push me inside. There was too little room to assist me out of the chair easily and safely. The wheelchair was too big and it was hard to maneuver it in such a confined place. Only with my strength to help could the aide succeed in lifting me out of the chair. The hazards involved when just one aide has to lift and assist a heavy patient out of an unstable wheelchair are enormous. Sometimes the patient falls and the aide gets the blame.

Being seated in this room was a revelation to say the least. It had a second door which led to another patient room, and I was apprehensive about the possibility of someone coming through it since it could not be locked for safety reasons. Right then, I knew that having the same lavatory for adjoining rooms should not be allowed. No amount of savings on construction costs justifies this humiliating and unnatural practice. This is abuse by regulation, one of the many kinds of degradations sponsored by regulatory agencies, developers, and designers of long term care facilities.

Supper finally arrived at my room and I was positioned next to my bed with the over-the-bed-table placed at my feet. A nurse placed my supper tray on it and stood by to be sure I could feed myself. She was most kind and made it clear that seconds could be had for the asking. Although I appreciated her advising me of this, I realized it would be an imposition to request additional food because there were so many patients who had to be spoonfed and I knew that when she left my side she would be assisting those people. It occurred to me that many residents may feel the same way and accept deprivation rather than disturb the busy staff.

I do not remember, exactly, what that first nursing home meal consisted of, but I *do* remember that it took a lot of complicated maneuvering to manipulate the cafeteria-style tray and dishes on the over-the-bed table, which was barely large enough to hold all the paraphernalia. Seated side-saddle in the wheelchair, with my leg extended in front of me, I had extreme difficulty getting positioned so that I could reach the food easily. Frankly, I began to feel that a good over-the-bed table would be one you could make disappear! All too frequently it was in my way.

Following supper, the balance of the evening was spent back in the lounge among the other patients. This was the only place I could go for a change of scenery and chance to smoke—a habit I had discontinued prior to admittance but readopted to combat my anxieties. Most importantly, it was the place where I could seek out other rational patients with whom I could converse and learn what they thought and felt. In sorrowful ways, I found it an extremely interesting room.

It was now time for my first contest with the TV set. One of my daily pleasures is watching the evening news, and I was looking forward to being updated on world events. At 6:30 the news program came on, but then something happened. A patient rolled her wheelchair up to the set and turned it to another channel. Remarks started flowing around the lounge from other patients: "Leave it alone!" "Take your hands off!" "Turn it back." "Don't touch it!" "Don't turn it back!" "I like that!" "Good!" "She shouldn't be in here!" Although I said nothing, I must admit that a speck of hostility toward the channel turner glowed within me.

Nine o'clock arrived and fatigue, induced principally by mental stress, came over me. I was looking forward to going to bed in order to escape from the setting I was in and to have a quiet opportunity to collect my thoughts.

A nurse named Rose asked if I would like to go to bed. When I told her I was tired, she pushed me back to my room and prepared the bed. Then she pushed me over to the sink and asked if I could wash myself. I told her I could and, as I soaped and cleansed my hands, she stayed by my side and ran her hand through my hair. She was very concerned about her unkempt alcoholic charge who was spending his first night in a home. I needed this human touch and I thought how beautiful it was for her to give it. Here was an example of the kindness that many nursing home staff members direct toward patients about which the general public seldom hears.

Rose took my pajamas from the bureau drawer and helped me into them and into bed. But the going-to-bed ritual was not yet over. It was time for recording my blood pressure, pulse, and respirations, and for administering my medication. A second nurse and a male orderly came in and stood at the foot of my bed while Rose conducted the physical examination. They seemed alarmingly curious—were they thinking how odd it was for such a relatively young person to be in their ward? It seemed obvious to me that they were silently questioning my presence. In order to ward off questions that might cause me to fumble and perhaps divulge my secret, I closed my eyes. Finally, they went away. Rose then gave me a pill for my minor stomach complaint and a capsule to make me sleep. The medication to induce sleep was not needed because I was fatigued, but since it was prescribed to help me get through the ten days, I swallowed it anyway. "Have a good night's sleep," Rose said as she turned out my bedside lamp, lifted up the bedside railings, forcefully set them in place, and walked away.

As I lay in bed, I consciously and deliberately analyzed the experience I was going through to learn how it feels and what it means for newly admitted patients to go to bed for the first time in a nursing home. Many nursing home patients are thinking people and I thought, "How incredible it is that all committed people go through this ritual knowing that this is probably the last bed in which they will sleep." I was aware, of course, that I was actually rehearsing an event that would, in all probability, become a real one later on. I knew that I would never forget this experience and would carry it with me for the rest of my days. A feeling of panic made me think I had, in fact, gone too far and should, perhaps, get out of bed, get my clothes, and go home. However, by reminding myself that I was only conducting an experiment, I was able to muster the fortitude to accept what was happening. Rose had helped a great deal by being so kind-hearted. From her I learned that *giving support to patients at bedtime the first night is one of the most important responsibilities the nursing home nurse has.*

The snaps and clicks of the bedrails still echoed. I was now safe from a tumble out of bed and secure for the night. A feeling of total dependence merged with a feeling of being trapped. I was now completely subject to the system and had to rely on the call button to satisfy my needs.

If I had really been disabled, it would have taken an enormous amount of effort to get out of bed with those railings up.

The easiest way out was over the footboard at the bottom of the bed. I recalled that patients had tried that in the homes I had administered, and that injuries had sometimes resulted. Panic, loneliness, and fear of confinement, I speculated, must cause patients to do that.

I could see my portion of the room by the light coming in from the corridor. On my right, four feet from my bed, was a wall. To my left, the only window was blocked from my view by the drawn divider curtain that separated Mr. Johnson's bed from mine. Five feet from the foot of my bed was another wall. Everything looked strange. Looking straight up, I could see only the ceiling, the walls, and the drawn curtain. The curtain track fixed to the ceiling seemed to be the border that designated "my" space—the only space I could really call my own, the only place for "privacy." Here was the place I would look forward to occupying each night to think about my family, count off the days, and meditate. I thought about all the other patients who most certainly lie in bed and think about their predicament too. I felt so alone. How fortunate I was to have the physical dexterity to reach that call button. How desperate seriously disabled patients must feel if they cannot signal for help.

I soon became aware of a decided indentation in the mattress made by those who had occupied the bed before me. The contours of the indentation did not fit my body. Morbid thoughts entered my mind. I wondered how many people had died in that bed. Certainly, I thought, other newly admitted patients must have similar thoughts and feelings. That *death image* pressed in the mattress has got to be a reminder of the temporary nature of one's occupation of a nursing home bed.

The first day had taught me a great deal. In particular, I now understood how newly admitted patients feel, and how great their need is for empathy, compassion, and understanding.

5

The Next Nine Days

During the remainder of my stay, I took as many notes as possible on my experiences. I was particularly interested in how influencing factors in the home such as applied public health standards, the design of the facility, and staff-patient relationships might inhibit patients from satisfying their needs. To gain an understanding of residents' lives, I projected myself into every situation possible.

I soon found that I was not only observing, but was reacting to, the historically founded procedures and perpetuated operational policies of the typical nursing home. The drama taking place before me was the same as in the institution I administered. In fact, it was common to most nursing homes—little has happened over the years to change old habits and customs. Each day was a replay of the day before. Mealtimes were the same, the hours set aside for use of the arts and crafts room were regulated, and the nurses administered medications and treatments on schedule as prescribed by attending physicians. I, like the other residents, spent my time conforming to the order programmed for us.

The Shower

Probably one of the most memorable experiences I had took place on the second day, when I was required to have a shower. The procedure involved was the same that all but the most severely disabled patients go through in most every home. It started one morning with the announcement by the nurse in charge that it was my time for a shower. Some minutes later, a rolling shower chair was pushed into my room. I was then undressed with the assistance of a pretty young nurses' aide and helped onto the special chair. A flannel blanket was wrapped around me, leaving only my head protruding. Feeling quite strange and embarrassed, I was spun around and moved with dispatch out of my room past some nurses and patients, down the corridor, and into the shower stall.

This room resembled a six- by ten-foot closet. It was typical of shower areas in nursing homes. It had no windows and the walls were ceramic-tiled. It had a wood bench at one end. Seated in the chair, I was placed under the shower head and the blanket was flicked off me. I felt humiliated. It was all such an undignified procedure. I thought, why do architects design shower rooms like this, and why hasn't someone in the nursing home field developed a more dignified procedure? I recalled the many patients in the homes I had administered who resisted, resented, and feared this degrading system.

My shower aide was most attentive and gracious. I marveled that she, and many others who care for disabled older people, would assume that kind of responsibility and do it with such kindness. I believe that only very compassionate and dedicated people are willing to provide this kind of service to others. Being aware of the many types of infirmity that patients in the typical nursing home have, my admiration and respect for nurses' aides increased.

Religious Observances

Sunday, my fourth day, was the one day of the week that was special because the routine could be broken by religious observances. It was the time when patients dressed in their finery and hoped for visitors. I observed many of my colleagues enjoying their callers. For those who did not have visitors, and there were many, just seeing people from the outside was a diversion from the usual boring routine, and they were pleased when strangers stopped to pass the time of day for a few moments or simply smiled and said hello.

Since the facility had both an in-house chaplain and an interdenominational chapel, some of the patients went to religious services. Homes do not ordinarily have these accommodations. Construction regulations do not require a chapel, nor are clergymen's salaries permitted as a legitimate operating expense under federal programs. Only institutions which underwrite these costs from profits provide such amenities. Where they do not exist, patients are discouraged from identifying with their former houses of worship. Many of those confined to nursing homes were once very involved spiritually, but were forced to abandon their religious ties upon admittance. I knew from experience that churches of all denominations, in all communities, make only token efforts to overcome this separation problem.

The Social Worker

Monday, day five, was my day to see the social worker. Her mission was to review my entire history and determine if she could help me resolve any personal difficulties. Regrettably, I had to be evasive and uncooperative in response to her questions. After just a few minutes, it became obvious to her that I didn't wish to talk, and she went back to her office.

This lady was the only social service person working in the entire large facility. The rules and regulations do not require more. Yet, because there were so many patients who needed all kinds of help, I knew she was overextended. How could a single person in her capacity effectively serve the entire home? It was impossible for her to explore all the concerns of patients and their families. Obviously, only major problems received her time and attention. Other needs, some important and meaningful, had to go unmet.

The Wheelchair

During my entire stay, I tried to analyze the elements that were affecting my life. The wheelchair I occupied, for instance, gave me mobility and a sense of independence because it allowed me to move about from place to place. However, I found that it was not the easiest thing to use. It required strength and good coordination. People with limited arm use due to strokes and other limitations, I observed, found it particularly hard to utilize. Some people who were confined to the device stayed in their rooms rather than expend their energy in moving about.

Although a wheelchair offers mobility and a little independence, architectural barriers in the traditional nursing home environment limit travel in it. Like other patients, I managed to bump into objects and an occasional door frame. Having a leg extended made it particularly difficult to use.

I learned by experience that it is a lot easier to roll a wheelchair over linoleum or tile floors than over carpeting. Passing over carpet moulding was particularly hard. Some patients, the disabled and weak, got stuck and had to summon assistance to help them maneuver over that bumpy edging.

Wheelchairs have many other disadvantages. The brake mechanisms, for example, are not easy to manipulate. One has to be keen witted to set and release the holding levers. Many patients push the wheels manually rather than use the special discs designed for that purpose. Their hands get dirty, as mine did from time to time, and pick up bacteria from the floor, so eating with contaminated fingers is a distinct possibility.

The Lack of Freedom

Traditional nursing home environments are very incarcerating. They restrict freedom in a variety of ways. Patients may be permitted to move about at will, but there are few places for them to go. My usual routine was to roam the corridor or move back and forth between my room and the single lounge in my ward. When one is situated on an upper floor as I was, without ready access to the outside and without unrestricted use of the elevator, there is no sense of being free. Going outdoors or to a distant part of the facility requires special permission and extra attention from the nurses. Because the staff is busy, patients do not ask for "favored" treatment. Although one could say that this particular freedom deprivation is, in part, a self-administered one, it is really induced by the nature of the environment and the systems employed.

The Bedroom

I spent part of my time analyzing the room in which I lived. It was designed to satisfy public health regulations and, like ordinary hospital rooms, it was small. There was very little space in which to keep personal possessions. Privacy was nonexistent; conversations were never private. When visitors came to see my room partner, Mr. Johnson, I either took part in the conversation or left the room. This was standard procedure for all the patients who were assigned to double rooms. There was no clock or calendar in my room and I found it very unsettling not to know the time of day or be sure of the date. In addition, there was no telephone, TV, or radio to stimulate my interest in the outside world. These standard and accepted deprivations, I speculated, must contribute to patients' mental regression and lethargy.

The Feeling of Dislocation

Finding my room after leaving it was not an easy task. I could not always recall which doorway led into my room and I frequently started to enter the wrong one thinking it was mine. Actually, this should not have been a problem because the home was attractively decorated and each room had different colored drapes and decor. Mine was predominantly blue. Unfortunately, no one told me I had the only blue room and I failed to research the others to make this determination myself. A black sweater and book that I left laying on the top of my bureau was the clue for me to realize I had located my bedroom. Since they were my property, I was then certain I was headed into the right place. Personal objects, I learned, are vitally important to help patients maintain their sense of orientation in nursing homes.

The Lounge

The experience of sitting in the lounge with the other patients was very saddening. This room was frequently occupied by a cross section of the patient population. Some would be parked there by the staff so that they would be out of their rooms and have some contact with others. As a consequence, the confused, the disoriented, and the incontinent were lumped together with mentally alert and rational people. This condition caused an abnormal amount of anxiety and frustration for the mentally competent. The nursing staff was also concerned and stressed over this arrangement. On one occasion a patient soiled the carpet just a few feet in front of me, and a nurse had to scrub it with soap and water and use a disinfectant to remove the feces. It is obvious that the floor plan of the facility, and the resultant lack of opportunity for suitable alternatives to sitting in that one lounge, fostered these abnormal and depressing conditions.

The Panic

On the sixth night, as I was sitting in the lounge, I suddenly panicked in that atmosphere and wanted to leave. Apparently the environment and the separation from my family was making me react this way. I went to a pay phone in the corridor, dialed my residence, and said to my wife, "This is too much. I don't think I can go through with it." She replied, "If you want to come home, I'll come and get you. If you want to stay, we are all with you." These words seemed to be what I needed to hear in order to gather my composure and muster the determination to go on with the experiment. Communication with my family was of vital importance to me. I needed to talk to someone close to me—someone who cared about me, not another "inmate" like myself. After calming down, I thought how likely it was that other people living in the home had similar feelings but, for a variety of reasons, could not call home. How anguishing that must be!

The Surrender

Peculiar things started to happen to my psyche on the day following this experience. I began to lose interest in what I was doing. It seemed that I had satisfied my curiosity and now only wanted to ride out the time until the ten days had gone by. It was no longer novel to be called by a different name. In fact, the identity that I had assumed when I was admitted now seemed to belong to me. There were moments when I thought I was there under legitimate circumstances and was a bona fide nursing home patient with justifiable physical complaints. Preoccupation with my family diminished. I was becoming displeased with things as they related to me as an individual. For example, I became somewhat annoyed at the environment and irritated when meals did not arrive in my room precisely on time. Apparently, the system had done its work on me. My true identity was being discarded. I was now reacting like an authentic patient and had surrendered my interest in viewing the nursing home environment in an objective sense.

The Leave-Taking

The ninth, and next to last, day was special because it demonstrated the altruistic nature of many nursing home employees. The staff was aware that I would soon leave them and they wanted to do something nice for me before I left. They arranged to have a nurse named Winnie take two other patients and me to a nearby ice-cream parlor to celebrate my discharge on the next day. The party came off as planned and I enjoyed the ice-cream, but Winnie, kind and sincere, did not realize how difficult this excursion was for me.   I was troubled by an impulse to tell her who I really was and what   I was doing, and to apologize. In the event, I managed to hold onto my thoughts, and we returned to the nursing home as arranged.

The last day finally came. My discharge was ready and my friend arrived to take me home. Before leaving, I visited around the facility to say goodby to as many patients and staff members as I could. Each time I expressed a final greeting, my guilt feelings multiplied. It was a very perplexing experience. I felt like an imposter, but I was sincerely indebted to everyone. While I had become more aware of the deficiencies of the traditional nursing home environment, I had been overwhelmingly impressed with the dedication of the staff and the work they did.

When I finally got into the car, my friend said, "Where do you want to go?" I answered, "Take me to the nearest good restaurant. I must go where there is a lot of normal activity—the last ten days have almost been too much to bear!" What I had seen and learned would be on my mind for the remainder of my life, but at the moment I wanted a dramatic change.

My experience had been multidimensional: 1) that of a patient; 2) that of an imposter; and, 3) that of an intensely involved analyst. My perceptions of nursing home life had been altered. I had become emotionally involved with the lives of patients and felt compelled, more than ever, to try to change the dehumanizing and depriving environments of nursing homes.

6

Analyzing the Traditional Nursing Home Environment

Character Of The Nursing Home Environment

The homes I administered represented the traditional kinds of facilities. They functioned within the framework of standard operating guidelines and, therefore, had all the built-in influences which can cause patients to be deprived and sometimes have degrading experiences.

After being a patient, I became more and more bothered about how and why sad things happen in homes. My reflections on my experience made me question the effectiveness of the whole geriatric system because I had come to realize that many of the deprivations levied upon patients are excessive. In fact, I felt guilty at having been a part of such a desperate scene and disappointed that I had not done more to correct it. I wondered why nursing home conditions are like they are, how they got that way, and why care standards that were inaugurated so many years ago were still in place.

It is clear to me that the basic reason for deficient nursing home care lies in the conflict *between the purpose for which these facilities should exist and the regulatory system used to operate them.* First and foremost, these institutions should be *homes,* with living arrangements which permit patients to enjoy life as much as possible. Their environments should at least allow residents to have privacy and freedom and be able to satisfy their other basic human needs to the fullest. This is not the case, however, because construction standards and patient care modes have been standardized to accommodate stereotyped ideas about older people and their needs.

Nursing homes are designed and built according to specifications developed for acute care hospitals. Anyone who has been a patient in that type of institution and then visited a nursing home would recognize the similarities. The ward "corridor," with patient rooms on either side and a single sitting room or lounge, is a takeoff on medical institutions. In fact, the environments are so much alike that if operating and laboratory services were added to homes they could readily function as general hospitals. By copying established medical models, nursing homes offer little in their environments to indicate they are places for living and not places to experience illness and eventual death. They are anything but homes.

The Physical Environment

As part of my effort to uncover environmental factors which might deprive patients, all of the rules and regulations governing the operation of nursing homes were reviewed. Requirements having a direct bearing on patients' quality of life were then correlated with the basic human needs identified in Chapter 3.

The Size of Patients' Rooms

Guideline #8.2-A of the *Federal Regulations for the Construc-*

tion of Long Term Care Facilities is the standard which regulates the size of rooms in all of today's nursing homes. For patients' rooms it specifies:

> Maximum room capacity shall be four patients. . . . Minimum room areas, exclusive of toilet rooms, closets, lockers, wardrobes, alcoves, or vestibules, shall be 100 square feet in single-bed rooms and 80 square feet per bed in multi-bed rooms.

Some state health agencies enforce regulations with minimum floor area requirements slightly larger than the federal guidelines. Massachusetts, for example, stipulates that the floor space must be at least 90 square feet per bed in multi-bed rooms and 125 square feet for single rooms. The homes I administered conformed to the latter specifications. In either case, however, the space suggested per patient is inadequate. People cannot move about freely in such close quarters.

While a patient, my two-bed room was always crowded (90 percent of nursing home beds are in multi-bed rooms). There was hardly enough space for me to maneuver my wheelchair in such a confined area. A variety of objects were in my way when I tried. Of my 90 square feet of space, the bed occupied 30, the bedside stand used up four, an over-the-bed table took up six, a floor lamp required two, a chair needed eight, and my half of the bureau absorbed about nine square feet. The total square footage for these pieces of furniture was approximately 59 square feet. This left the equivalent of 31 square feet, or an area representing less than six by six feet, for ambulating, moving my wheelchair, and keeping miscellaneous personal belongings. My wheelchair alone took up an additional nine square feet. Not included in these calculations is the floor space used up by the hanging privacy curtains or other pieces of special equipment which might be needed from time to time, and the space occupied by inward opening doors.

The usable floor area in patient rooms is distributed around the beds, which are positioned against one wall. There is hardly enough room to turn a wheelchair around. Nurses have to drag and sometimes lift the patients, chair and all, when they move them about or in and out of the rooms. The space allotment does not even allow for meaningful patient exercise, and the over-the-bed table and other objects present tripping hazards to those who try to walk. The condition is particularly dangerous to people who are unsteady on their feet or have difficulty walking. It should not be surprising, therefore, that nursing homes have numerous incidents where patients trip, fall, and sustain fractures. Sadly, the regulated standards which have induced such space limitations have made patients' rooms very dangerous and extremely incarcerating.

Even though the single-room space requirements are somewhat larger per patient (100 square feet), they also are pitifully small. Patients need to have extra things—an extra chair, a small table, a television set, or other personal effects. With just a few additional belongings, people living in private rooms are left with little extra space for walking or moving about in a wheelchair.

Nursing home construction regulations mandate a minimum of three feet between beds, three feet between beds and a lateral wall, and a four foot passageway at the foot of the beds. These specifications are totally inadequate. A wheelchair alone is three feet wide. With the footrests extended it is over four feet long. Again, there is not enough floor space to permit the rotation of a wheelchair. While a patient, I had to roll my chair backwards to get along the side of my bed. In fact, I had to start rolling myself backwards in the corridor outside of my room in order to end up positioned next to the bed. This feat was rarely accomplished without bumping into something that blocked my way. As can be expected, some patients stay in their rooms rather than fight the obstacle course and play the role of wheelchair jockeys.

A four-foot passageway at the foot of the beds is unreasonably small. It does not allow patients to go by one

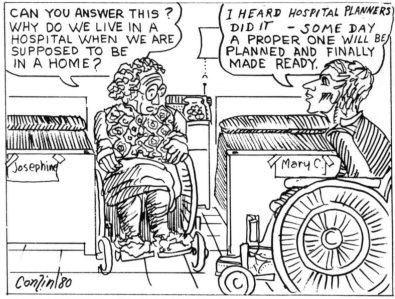

THE HOSPITAL ENVIRONMENT.........

another without some risk. In a home I administered, a patient ambulating in this passageway tripped over another's foot, fell down, and fractured his hip. And, of course, it is impossible for two wheelchair patients to pass in such close quarters. It is common to witness patients having arguments or colliding in their chairs at the foot of a bed. Sometimes they are seen rolling their chairs back and forth, bumping and pushing each other's vehicle because they are angry over being interfered with.

The Systems and Procedures

The internal systems, procedures, and methods of delivering care in nursing homes also emulate the hospital sector. Both systems were originated by public health regulatory agencies for the sole purpose of satisfying patients' physical-medical needs without regard to other needs. For example, the three-times-a-day nurse charting routine (not always necessary), the daily monitoring of vital signs, the bathing procedures, and the nurse duty assignments all originate from standard medical traditions. How these procedures affect the patients' daily lives has never been a serious consideration of health planners. Very little, if anything, has been carried over from hospitals to respect the patients' quality of life. As a result, many social and psychological patient needs go unmet and lifestyles necessary for acutely ill people are prescribed for every resident. Many who could live meaningful lives are forced to be dependent and conform to old and stultifying routines.

Most nursing home patients are not sick. They may be disabled to some degree, but generally they feel well. As a patient and as an administrator, I have made a point of asking patients how they feel. They almost always respond by saying they feel fine. Most, no matter what their disabilities, do not have pain or discomfort to cause them to say otherwise. Yet the physical environment and operational procedures are designed for acute care hospitals, which care for the sick and do not accommodate those who are well. Because of this, it is the alert and well patients who suffer the greatest deprivations in nursing homes. They live in environments incompatible with their needs and have only meager opportunities to live private, meaningful, and peaceful lives.

Hardships Imposed by the Level of Care System

As you may recall from Chapter Two, the level of care classifications are: Intensive Nursing and Rehabilitative Care Facility (also called Extended Care Facility)—Level I; Skilled Nursing Facility—Level II; Supportive or Intermediate Care Facility—Level III; and Resident Care Facility or Rest Home—Level IV. As previously indicated also, a home may have one or more of these designations. It is important to realize, however, that all multi-level homes must be sectioned off by units, commonly referred to as wards. It is the patient's diagnosis and prognosis that qualifies him or her for residency in one of these sections. The essential difference between classifications is the amount of nursing time and rehabilitation therapies alloted to the patients.

The level of care system is important to understand because of the impact it has on the patients' ability to satisfy their needs for freedom and the exercise of their decision-making powers. First of all, the number of homes available for occupancy are limited. For example, an older person may wish to live in a favored home but cannot because that facility was designated differently from what his or her diagnosis requires. I have known of a number of cases where man and wife lived in different institutions because they did not have the same classifications. I've also seen husbands and wives living in the same facility but separated by assignments to different units or wards.

The theory behind the earmarking of patients for specific kinds of service is that it minimizes the cost of care and at the same time delivers quality care. The fact of the matter is, it is discriminatory, causes unforgivable hardships to patients and their families, is wasteful of taxpayers' money, and sponsors substandard care. It places the nursing emphasis on medical needs and devalues the importance of serving the patients' social, psychological, and daily living needs. That the anxiety and stress induced by the system might contribute to residents' physical and mental decline is overlooked. Certainly, patients who require specialized medical care will get the maximum available attention time regardless of what level of care they may be assigned to. Trained professional registered nurses know who should and who should not receive the benefit of their training. Having a regulated system to prorate care on the basis of nursing time in a nursing home is unnecessary. Nurse staffing should be based only on the number of patients residing in the facility, and should not be complicated by allocating it on the basis of medical needs.

That the level of care system is wasteful and costly is evidenced by the monitoring and clerical detail required to administer the program. Volumes of paperwork are done to keep track of the assigned classifications. Physicians spend hours and hours of their time reviewing patients' diagnosis just to be certain the physical conditions will warrant residence in a particular part of a home or a transfer to another facility. Special monitoring committees (case review and utilization review committees) and persons, including paid doctors, function to force transfers of patients from one level to another. For example, all Skilled and Intermediate nursing homes (Levels I, II, and III) are required by regulation to utilize these committees, on which it is necessary to have two physicians serving. Each doctor is paid $50 or more per hour. This alone represents an expenditure of millions of dollars per year.

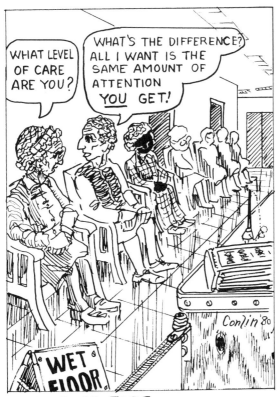

LEVELS OF CARE.....

Finally, the level of care system does not work because, as a rose is a rose, a nursing home patient is a nursing home patient. Their *quantity* of needs—medical, social, and others—and the *amount* of staff attention time required to service those needs is the same regardless of where they reside. The difference is a matter of which needs must be satisfied first. Patients whose medical needs are highest in order of priority require staff time to satisfy those needs first, along with staff service time to satisfy their social and psychological needs second. Persons who have fewer medical needs require staff time to satisfy their social and psychological needs first. In other words, the sum total of staff support time needed by each patient is the same regardless of the classification involved. Unfortunately, the level system prevents this from happening. It sponsors more staff attention time for patients living in Levels I and II and a lesser amount of staff time for those assigned to Level III. Consequently, many who have been classified as Level III patients and who need some assistance to participate in social activities, or who wish to exercise greater independence, receive less nursing attention than Level I and II patients.

My experience as a patient exposed me to the unnecessary hardships that level transfers place upon patients. Mr. Redd, one of the people with whom I became friendly, was informed one afternoon that he was going to be moved downstairs to another unit because his classification had changed from Level II to Level III. He said to me, "They're going to take my room away and give me one downstairs—I don't know anyone down there." Then he said, "I'm afraid—I see no need for this. What difference does it make to them where I am?" He was quite shaken by this truly unnecessary event. But he was moved anyway, because the regulations said he should be.

I also was directly involved with the level system. After being a Level II patient for four or five days, the director of nurses came to me and told me I was being considered for a transfer to a Level III bed. Although I knew it might be beneficial to my experiment to observe what happens in another section of the home, the idea of moving was hard to accept. I had become familiar with the routines and staff and felt secure. I didn't want to move. It meant I'd have to go through the process of getting familiar with the environment all over again and my anxieties would be increased. As it turned out, my room wasn't changed. I learned firsthand, however, that this aspect of nursing home life is unreasonably cruel. It demonstrated to me how medical modes supersede human values and cause unjustifiable hardships for patients.

Characteristics of the Nursing Home Patient

To learn *how* and *why* patients are deprived in nursing homes, it is essential to understand their physical and mental conditions. Their average age is approximately 82. Two-thirds are female and these patients are, on the average, a few years older than the male patients. Although most of them don't *feel* ill, they all have a variety of chronic and crippling disabilities. These include cardiovascular disease, arthritis, Parkinson's disease, arteriosclerosis, cerebral vascular accident (stroke), epilepsy, heart trouble, respiratory afflictions, fractures, diabetes, kidney failure, tumors, and other diseases associated with old age. About one-third of the cases are incontinent, having lost control over their bowel and/or bladder functions. There are also many who cannot ambulate or wash, bathe, dress, feed, or toilet themselves. Very few can do all of these things without staff assistance.

One outstanding fact, ignored by the medical system over the years, is the source of much of the neglect and deprivation suffered by nursing home patients. It is that the majority of the residents are mentally alert and rational and are not, by any means, senile. They know who they are, where they are, and the date, time, and place. The Senate Committee on Aging, in its *Failure in Public Policy* report of November, 1974, indicated that 45 percent of nursing home patients are *not* mentally impaired. Studies I conducted in the facilities I administered demonstrated that over half are mentally sound.

It is the rational patients who are most deprived and who suffer the greatest losses when admitted to a home. The operating systems are not designed to recognize or focus on them. They are the people who try hardest to cope with the environment, to maintain their independence, mental stability, and sense of dignity.

While a patient, I was very conscious of the plight of the rational patients. They were a lost group, obviously living in an environment which was unsuited to their needs. Many were in wheelchairs, some used walking aids, others had severely crippling disabilities, but they were mentally alert and it didn't seem right that they should have to spend most of their time among those who had mental afflictions and were illogical and disturbing. Some were even assigned to rooms where confused and disoriented patients also lived. It made no difference whether they were in their rooms, in the corridor, or seated in the lounge, there was no escape from the abnormal and depressing behavior of the irrational patients.

The current effort on the part of mental institutions to place many mentally disturbed patients in nursing homes is having a very depressing effect on alert residents. Their living conditions are being adversely affected and their anxieties are increasing. And this is happening even though many of the nursing home staff members are not trained to cope with patients who have serious mental illnesses.

I recall a conversation I had with a fellow patient while we were seated in the lounge one afternoon. One of the several confused ladies kept talking during a television program we were watching. He said to me, "That's terrible—they shouldn't let them come in here. All they do is make it worse for all of us!" I defended the lady by pointing out that she was not responsible and couldn't help herself. He responded in a somewhat disgusted voice, "You may be able to take it, but after you've been here awhile you'll lose your buttons, too!'' Actually, I should have agreed with him because I was also annoyed. She *did* interfere with our pleasure and there is no question but that there should have been a better place for her or a better place for us.

Because the lounge was a gathering place for every conceivable type of patient, those who were alert would not remain in it very long. When a disrupting person came in, one by one the rational people would leave and go back to their rooms. I also followed this pattern as it was too depressing to stay in the lounge when mentally afflicted people were also there. That many alert patients have to live in that kind of an environment for years is tragic. I came to wonder if irrationality didn't breed irrationality.

The Role of the Nursing Home Nurse

As a patient, I became more aware than ever of the work done by nurses and aides. They always have a multitude of supportive tasks to perform and very little time in which to complete them. On any given day or night they are under constant pressure by patients who need some kind of service. Although many of their tasks appear to be minor, all are demanding and time-consuming. They may be called upon to give someone a drink of water, to move a disabled person about, to take someone to the lavatory, or simply to talk to an individual who needs a friend. Mixed in with these responsibilities are the needs requiring skilled care and treatments for those who are seriously afflicted.

The nurses and aides care for a special group of older people having a variety of difficult and crippling disabilities. Care is given to those who are handicapped and need help to dress and undress. Many patients have to be spoonfed; sometimes, by necessity, three, four, or more have to be fed simultaneously by one nurse. Service has to be administered to the many who need assistance to walk, to incontinent people who require many changes of clothing and/or bedding each day and night, and to wheelchair cases needing an escort to travel about. Most difficult of all, the nursing staff must supervise and care for those who are mentally afflicted, disoriented, confused, disturbed, and noisy *besides* having one or more of the many disabilities associated with old age.

To work with nursing home patients, nurses are expected to have a multitude of qualities and skills. They must be kind, empathetic, compassionate, understanding, friendly, and be able to maintain their composure at all times. They are expected to set aside their own feelings, their personal hardships, and overlook the fact that they may not feel well themselves. In addition, they have to be familiar with all the patients' families, and be knowledgeable about current gerontological, social and psychological concepts applicable to the care of older people. And finally, to complete their qualifications, they must be psychiatric nurses, rehabilitation nurses, treatment nurses, and technicians skilled in the use of respirators, oxygen machines, and other specialized pieces of medical equipment. To add to all this, they cannot hope that the service they give will effect cures for the people they serve. Instead, their goals are to maintain the patients' well-being and make them as contented as possible until death approaches. When one considers all this, one may well come to the conclusion that nursing home nurses are more altruistic than those found in other parts of the medical field.

I have come to believe that the standard regulated nurse staffing patterns applied to nursing homes are inadequate and should be questioned. There are too many patient demands and too few staff members to satisfy the needs of all the patients, and the result is patient deprivation.

While I was a patient, and thinking about staffing patterns, I became conscious of the amount of attention time that was given to me. It was surprisingly little. In fact, **after** the fourth day, when I had progressed out of the wheelchair and had begun to ambulate independently, it was negligible. I estimated that the average amount of time that a nurse or other staff member was in direct contact with me was from five to ten minutes out of a 24-hour period. This may seem hard to believe, but when one considers the time patients sleep, the noncontact duties of the nurses, their break times, and the fact that it takes only seconds for staff members to deliver a food tray or hand medication to a patient, it is understandable why the time involved is so very little. This does not mean that the nursing staff is not busy because a great deal of their time is spent planning, preparing, and giving direct service for the more demanding patients. What it does indicate, however, is that by no means are nursing homes overstaffed.

There are deep-rooted misconceptions regarding the merits of nursing home nursing, some of them harbored by influential health professionals associated with acute care. Administering bedside care in a hospital setting to patients who are critically ill is often considered more glamorous and more indicative of nursing skills than other types of nursing. On the other hand, delivering care to people in long term facilities is thought to be less meaningful, less rewarding, and to call for fewer skills.

This characterization of long term nursing is frequently heard within the nursing home field itself. I've attended numerous long term care gatherings, training programs, and seminars, and have heard members of the medical profession misrepresent as minimal the needs of geriatric patients for professional nursing care. At one of these meetings I heard a nursing home owner, who was herself a nurse, downplay the importance of professional care. I vividly remember the term "baby sitters" being applied by a physician to the nursing staff of a facility I administered. His concept of the needs of nursing home patients had been distorted by his experience and absorption in acute care. That the quality of service delivered in homes depends upon skilled supervision and sound medical and psychological support, and that patients are dependent upon the staff for their every need, was not understood by him. He sincerely believed that the patients had insignificant or few unmet needs and that those they did have could be satisfied by a minimum number of unskilled personnel.

If, however, this professional practitioner had spent a whole day in a nursing home and had observed the staff at work and the desperate plight of the patients, his opinions would have altered. Unfortunately, the kind of bias exhibited by this doctor discredits nursing homes and fosters substandard care.

In order to show that the needs of nursing home patients are unique, that they require special nursing skills, and that the merits of long term nursing should not be judged on the basis of acute care needs, I made a comparative analysis of the duties and responsibilities of the two types of nursing. The results are shown in the following list.

A Comparison of Essential Nursing Responsibilities in Nursing Homes and Acute Care Facilities

Nursing Home Nursing	*Acute Care Nursing*
Patients are served for months and years.	Patients are served for days and weeks.
objective is to maintain the patients' well-being.	The objectives are cure oriented.
Nurses are skilled in serving patients who have diseases associated with old age.	Nurses are skilled in serving patients with acute illnesses.
The death experience is a certainty for every patient.	Most patients are discharged to their homes.
Nurses have had long lasting relationships with families at the time of death.	Nurse-family relationships, if any, were relatively short at time of a death.
Nurse substitutes as a family member.	Nurse does not usually substitute as a family member.

Nurse is involved with the patient's personal life.	Nurse does not get involved with the patient's personal life.
The patients are not cured.	Most patients experience a cure.
Emotional involvement with the patients is desirable and important.	Emotional involvement with the patients is discouraged.
High percentage of patients are dependent on nurses for their total needs.	Lower percentage of patients are dependent on nurses for their total needs.
The social and recreational needs of patients are a critical part of care.	The social and recreational needs of patients are either not significant or not very significant.
The percentage of incontinent patients is high.	The percentage of incontinent patients is low.
Many mentally afflicted patients are served.	Few mentally afflicted patients are served.
Service is given to many non-ambulatory patients.	Most patients are ambulatory or become ambulatory.
Nurses must be knowledgeable about gerontological concepts.	Nurse knowledge of gerontology is not as significant since it is not applicable to a large percentage of patients.
Physicians place heavy reliance on nurse judgement. (Inconsistent physician monitoring)	Physician reliance on nurse judgement not as great. (Frequent physician monitoring).

7

How the Author Perceived Residents' Needs Before, During, and After His Experience

The basic human needs listed in Chapter Three are discussed here in the order of priority that was given to them by the patients (see page 37).

Possessions: What Their Loss Means

After living in a typical nursing home room, I became very conscious of what space limitations mean to patients, and thought about the policies I had implemented in the homes I administered to overcome patients' space deprivations. I had always been concerned with the patients' needs for possessions. When people were admitted to the facility, I would talk to them, their families, and sometimes to the staff about the importance of permitting private property in the residents' rooms. I encouraged the use of television sets and radios, providing they didn't disturb others. Family photographs were encouraged, as was a personal upholstered chair (if space was available). I would counsel patients about their needs to have a little money at all times, but not too much because it might get mistakenly picked up by another inmate or a member of the staff, or even sent to the laundry in error. Patients and their families were also asked to supply clothing, but to be careful not to over-crowd the single wardrobe. Knitting equipment, writing materials, and bulletin boards were encouraged, too. I offered Scotch tape so greeting cards and pictures could be stuck on the doors and walls.

Another way I attempted to satisfy the patients' needs for possessions was to suggest to disabled people that they have their "own" wheelchair by using a marking device to print their names in large letters on the backrest so everyone would know who "owned" the chair. In these, and other ways, I conveyed the idea that the staff of the facility supported their having possessions. I believed that I was doing everything possible to help guests satisfy this basic need.

Now I realize that my possession policies were minuscule—just token expressions of goodwill. The magnitude of the patients' personal property deprivation is great and almost total. Patients want and need much more than I was giving them. As I sat among them and analyzed their plight, I could sense and empathize with their feelings after having left *all* of their worldly belongings behind them—furniture, sentimental artifacts, hanging pictures, plants, valuables such as jewelry, and most of their clothing. Except for the windowsill, the bedside stand, and the top of a shared bureau, there is little space in a patient's room for the display of pictures and other treasured things. Irrespective of the patients' prior lifestyles, being bereft of their property makes them seem destitute.

The many conversations I had with patients when *I* was a patient made me more sensitive to their possession losses. They would talk with pride about the house or apartment they used to have, and make such comments as, "I used to have a lot of things, but I don't have anything now—everything is gone!"

They yearned for the things they used to have, and were now missing—forever.

I vividly recall a conversation I had with Mr. Greene, one of the patients. He told me a little of his life history—how he had been a machinist and had had a nice cottage, and how he had raised and educated his children. To conclude his story, he said to me, "When you are working and making good money, have your own home, raise a family, you never expect that one day you will have to give it all up and come into a place like this!" Then he said disgustedly, "Here you have nothing!"

Storage spaces and drawers for essential garments are sorely lacking in homes. This condition, like the many others which deprive patients, are underwritten by nursing home operational

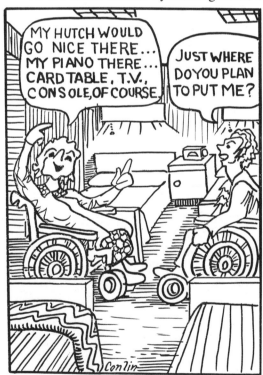

POSSESSIONS . . . .

standards. The opportunity for storing a meaningful selection of clothes is severly limited. Patients wear the same outer garments over and over again and the same shoes day in and day out. Winter clothing is not usually found in wardrobes because there is not enough room. Seldom do you see men wearing suits or having a selection of suits hanging in their closets.

It can be argued that nursing home patients do not need much clothing since they do not go anywhere. This is not a valid argument because when people lose most of their cherished garments they lose their sense of self. Dressing neatly and having a variety of attire is a means of maintaining self-respect and dignity. Being admitted to a home should not mean that one has to automatically adopt a stereotyped lifestyle or lock-step dress.

Some patients do try to maintain their sense of dignity by dressing neatly. They are usually strong characters who were at one time economically secure and accustomed to wearing good clothes. The men stand out because of a suit coat, vest, or tie that they wear over and over again, and the women by an expensive dress, now old, or a favorite piece of tasteful, inexpensive jewelry.

I remember Mr. McDonald, a man of Scottish origin who was a patient in the home where I worked. He had *one* suit and a Scotch plaid tie, both of which he wore day after day. His suit and tie made him stand out among the other patients in the facility and attracted frequent compliments from the staff. It was his way of preserving his individuality. It seemed sad to many of the staff members, however, that he didn't have several suits in his wardrobe so he could hear kind words about them also.

The kind of problems that patients have over the lack of storage space in their rooms can be illustrated by something that happened to Mr. McDonald. He had a bagpipe which he liked to play occasionally. Since there was no place to store it, he kept it in a corner of his room, where it was exposed to handling by anyone living or working in his unit. One day it was broken. He claimed it had been mishandled by another patient. To protect the instrument, his son removed it from the facility. It was never returned and Mr. McDonald never played his bagpipe again. The removal of personal and cherished possessions for protective reasons is standard operating procedure in many nursing homes.

Patients' Families and the Nursing Home Environment

I had always considered it important for patients to have intimate relationships with their families and consistent visits from them. What I did about this, however, was traditional and derivative in nature. I viewed families as being motivated to visit the home and believed they would do so without special efforts on the part of the nursing home. I did not fully understand that I should be giving higher priority to family needs and helping them in more meaningful ways to cope with the very saddening experience of having a loved one in the facility.

Although many homes follow hospital procedure and restrict visiting hours, this was not true of the institutions I administered. That mode is adopted to minimize visitor interference and prevent visitors from observing how patient care is delivered. The institutions where I worked had open visiting hours to encourage visitations throughout the day and evening. I was proud of the work done by the nursing staff and liked to have the community see what they did. This policy gave me greater control over the activities taking place in the wards because family members were asked to express their observations and concerns to me. In this way, I could adopt measures to correct the failures of our systems. My staff appreciated this policy, too, because they believed that responding to family questions would help them improve their care methods. It also gave the nurses and aides a greater opportunity to know the patients' next of kin, something that is vitally important in the delivery of long term care.

Aside from having open visiting hours, the social service and other departments carried out all the customary family-oriented procedures. For example, provisions were made for emergency visits at times of crisis. A cup of coffee or tea, a snack, or a full-course meal would be offered visitors when they were at the bedside of their loved ones during an emergency. From time to time a social worker would phone family members and ask them to visit, to bring something the patients wanted, or to attend special activity programs. In addition, the patients' next of kin could purchase meals at a reasonable price and were urged to have lunch or dinner in the home. Notices of special events were posted on the bulletin boards to encourage families to attend concerts and other events held in the home.

After studying the patients' needs for family, my perspective on the problem changed. I was made aware that I should do more and that the separation of my guests and their relatives is far greater than I had known. I learned that the traditional nursing home presents a "hostile environment," which, despite the efforts of my staff, discouraged visitations. That the environment is hostile is evidenced by the standard architectural design of the facilities. The multi-bed rooms that mix alert patients with those who are disoriented, the crowded lounges, the lack of privacy, and the occasional unpleasant odors, all present a depressing and oppressive scene.

There are other factors, too, which act as deterrants to regular visits by families. There is little in the way of accommodations for children who come into the home with their parents. They have no chance to visit Grandma or Grandpa alone. Quite frequently their presence is disturbing to other patients and they are told to be quiet. It is common for them to become impatient and be sent by their parents to the lobby to wait. Generally, they ask to be taken home and succeed in bringing Mom and Dad with them.

Freedom—Why Patients Lose It

The matter of patients' need for freedom has not received much attention in long term care literature or in staff educational programs. Significantly, neither have I heard the subject discussed among nursing home inspectors during my 16 years as an administrator. Freedom for patients is something that is ignored.

I had always claimed, and I'm sure other administrators have claimed, that the people admitted to homes have opportunities to move about freely and do as they wish. When new patients were brought in, I usually implied that, within reason, they could go wherever they wanted, when they wanted, and do what they wanted. This is part of the psychology of lightening the trauma of coming into a home. There is a difference, however, between saying something will happen and actually having it happen. Unfortunately, what is supposed to happen regarding patients' freedom to move about just does not happen.

Too many inhibiting factors are present in the traditional nursing home environment to permit true freedom. Actually, patients are virtual prisoners. Their freedoms are curbed by the physical environment, the outmoded care systems and procedures, and the regulated limited number of the nursing staff. The severely disabled are particularly confined because they do not have the capacity to move about independently. They spend hours, days, and weeks in their wards with almost no chance to go outside. This fact is verifiable simply by observing the activity taking place on the grounds around almost any nursing home. Few patients are seen outside during comfortable weather. For every one who is out, 10, 15, or more are held inside.

The fundamental responsibility for this condition rests with the federally sponsored construction standards for homes. No provisions are made to force the development of appropriate patient areas such as walkways, patios, exercise courses, gardens, or picnic grounds around the facilities. Also contributing are unknowledgeable and unempathetic developers who, while formulating construction plans, trade off construction of external amenities in favor of what they believe to be more important needs within the facilities.

One need only look at a typical nursing home ward to appreciate how many freedom limitations exist there. There is always a long corridor with rooms on either side. Only one lounge is available to patients where they may go for a change of scenery. Those who can move about independently are seen going back and forth from their rooms, to the corridor, to the lounge, and back to their rooms again. This is the customary extent of the freedom patients have to relieve boredom and alter the repetitive routines of the day.

Of course, homes do have other areas for patients' use, such as activity rooms, dining rooms, and sometimes a place designated as a chapel. The use of these areas, however, are, by necessity, most always limited. The greater number of patients

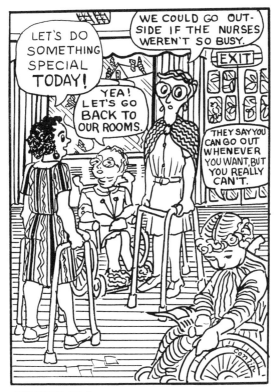

FREEDOM . . . .

must eat at their bedsides at prescribed moments. Time slots are usually alloted to the patients for visitations to the other places. Unfortunately, many people have to depend upon staff to escort them when leaving their wards. Usually there are not enough staff members available to accommodate everyone.

One of the most depriving aspects of nursing home life is the loss of patients' contact with the world beyond the walls of the institution. The opportunity for them to be part of the community is almost nil. This was made clear to me when I was a patient and observed groups of my colleagues frequently gathering at the large lounge windows to view the activities taking place on the streets in the distance. The more able people would reminisce and talk about the streets and buildings and experiences they had had in the past. Occasionally, confused people would be placed at the windows by the staff so they too could see the view. How tantalizing, I thought. I had the feeling as they stared through the glass that they were looking back, reaching out, and wishing, in their confused way, that they were somewhere else.

While in the lounge one day, I overheard a disturbing verbal interchange between two patients. After gazing out of the window for a few seconds, one of them turned and said to the other, "What are we doing here?" The sad reply was, "Waiting to be called!" How true it was. Admittedly, that is the regulated purpose of nursing home life.

On another day, a second incident occurred which focused on the same problem and gave me a deeper insight about patients' need for freedom. Again it happened in the vicinity of the lounge windows. A conversation was taking place among several people about going outside. One patient alluded to the fact that the administrator and staff members had indicated they were free to do so. Mr. Russell, one of the more independent and alert people said, "They say you can go out, but you really can't. If you want to go, you have to ask permission; then someone has to watch you; even then you can't go unless you have the doctor's permission." Other voices chimed in and one asked sardonically, "You mean the warden?" Then a humorous individual, the one who used a walker he called his horse, said, "He's the vet." Speaking about the nurses, the discussion ended with the comment, "They're too busy and have too much to do to let you go out." Never before had I fully realized the extent to which the patient's freedom is sacrificed. It is evident that the care systems are geared to satisfy the patients' survival needs and that other needs, due to the systems' deficiencies, go unattended.

The Need for Privacy

Privacy is something that is practically nonexistent in homes. Unless a resident has a private room, there just isn't any. Those who are in multi-bed accommodations, and that is 85 to 95 percent of the home population, move to obscure corners, wait for their roommate to leave, or visit the lavatory to find solitude. To speak of privacy existing in a nursing home is absurd.

In the past, I paid little attention to this need. It's a subject that is avoided by administrators when discussing nursing home life with patients and their families. It is as if loss of privacy is an accepted thing and should be expected. In a subconscious way, it is understood that nursing homes are not intended to provide such a luxury. What this deprivation might mean to the many rational patients is deliberately disregarded.

To create an illusion of privacy, homes, by regulation, provide hanging curtains which can be drawn around the beds to close them off from the view of people passing by. In this way, patients can at least go unseen when they are undressing or be cloistered when they are seriously ill. It is a system or procedure that has been inherited from hospitals, justified by the rationale that what is good enough for people in acute care is, ipso facto, good enough for nursing home residents.

The patients' want and need of privacy can be appreciated by watching how they manipulate this curtain. They will frequently pull it alongside their beds just far enough to block

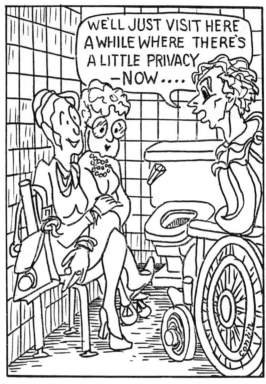

PRIVACY . . . .

their sight of the person in the next bed. In this way, they are able to separate themselves from their neighbor. This may be fine for the individual situated next to the window, but the poor souls farthest from it are closed off from a view of the outside. My bed was one of these and I spent every night and a good part of every day shut off from the bed next to mine and from the outside view.

This arrangement is a source of many conflicts in homes. Patients get into arguments over who has control over the use of the divider screens. Numerous complaints are made to the nurses and administrators by those who are frustrated because they are being closed in or being stopped from positioning the curtains to have a little privacy. I found this condition to be one of the major reasons many patients would like to have a private room.

Miss Smith, a patient in a facility I administered, typified the hardships and unhappiness caused by the curtain arrangement. She lived in a two-bed room. Her roommate, a lady of very strong character, had the bed next to the window and wanted constant isolation. She insisted that the screen be drawn between the beds at all times. Miss Smith resented being shut off from the rest of the room, but no sooner would she remove the barrier than her roommate would replace it. As a result, Miss Smith lived under continual stress and would get frequent asthmatic attacks. The nursing staff had to mediate between them daily in efforts to settle the issue. On several occasions, Miss Smith summoned me for help. When I visited her she would cry and plead with me to stop the continuous closing of the screen. Ultimately, she had to be moved to another room to resolve the problem. The staff and I knew, however, that the next person to occupy Miss Smith's former place would undergo the same frustrating experience.

Multi-bed rooms have many other disadvantages. For example, conversations which take place within them are seldom private. Visitors cannot talk without being overheard and are denied intimate family-patient interaction and communication. I recall the day when I was visiting an 89-year-old lady, someone I thought was the most beautiful person in the world—my mother. She said to me, "Whenever your father comes to see me he spends most of his time talking to someone else!" To overcome this kind of a predicament, family members are often seen pushing their relatives in wheelchairs, or walking with them up and down the corridors, or sitting with them in obscure places because they have a need to be removed from others and be free to talk in private. The total inconvenience of all this makes one question the merit of the nursing home standards which sponsor multi-bed rooms.

The lack of privacy has a conforming influence on patients. It induces in them a loss of spirit to live independent lives. Their daily experiences, and sometimes their confidential topics of conversations, become shared with the general population of the facility. Personal matters, particularly diagnostic information and physical complaints, end up as interesting subjects for discussion groups. Individual lifestyles cannot be preserved, for no matter what the patients' modes of living were before coming into the institution, they are forced to capitulate and live fragmented and nonconfidential lives. Individual characters and personalities become compressed and moulded into one model.

The Environmental Influences that Take away Patients' Independence

One of the primary objectives of a well-run home is to encourage patients to maintain maximum independence. Most nurses and aides want this for them and foster it as much as they can. When residents take the initiative and satisfy their own needs, it reduces the workload of the staff and saves valuable service time. The benefits of promoting self-reliance for activities of daily living, i.e., teaching patients how to dress themselves, groom themselves, feed themselves, maintain their own personal hygiene, and function at their maximum potential, is something that is stressed at inservice training programs.

I had always believed that independence was being encouraged in homes and that patients fought hard to preserve it. I thought, too, that nurse understaffing might be beneficial in that it fostered patients' self-reliance. Now I have come to realize that the forces operating in homes, i.e., insufficient nurse coverage and environmental factors, are actually counter to the attainment of independence. In fact, the systems used and the physical characteristics of the facilities cause dependence. Patients learn soon after admittance that the best way to get their share of staff attention is to become dependent.

It is the more disabled and medically demanding people who receive the most amount of nursing time. Those who may need just a little help to do for themselves cannot readily solicit assistance. Rather than be bothersome, they forgo making what they perceive as unreasonable demands and wait for staff attention. In the interim, they adopt alternative ways of satisfying their needs. For example, those who need just a little help to put on their shoes compromise by wearing slippers, those who may need minor support to get out of their chairs will stay seated by their beds, and those who require a bit of help to dress will stay in their night clothes. By so doing, they surrender to the system and accept the staff's perception of their needs. Consequently, *it is the people who have potential for independence who are most deprived.*

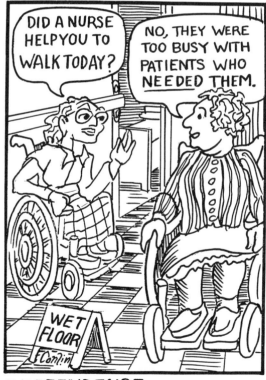

INDEPENDENCE . . . .

The design and physical layout of homes play a major part in preventing patients from functioning at their maximum independence level. Typical resident rooms are so congested that freedom of movement is severely restricted. This is particularly true for wheelchair patients. They often need a helping hand to move a bed, chair, or over-the-bed table which prevents them from traveling out of their rooms. I had experience with this while I was a wheelchair "patient." Furniture and equipment in the room was most always in my way. I had the strength to maneuver around these blockades but I observed others who would stay in their rooms until a nurse happened to come along.

It is rare that elderly patients will beat the nursing home system and win out in the struggle to preserve their independence. This did happen, however, to a courageous lady living in a facility I administered. The incident was one of the most joyful and pleasing experiences I ever had during all of my time as a nursing home administrator. I will call the person involved Mrs. Jones. In earlier years she had been a shrewd businesswoman who owned a profitable commercial establishment which was still in business while she was a patient. She had kept her apartment, to which she expected to return.

Mrs. Jones was 68 years old. She had one son, who was responsible for her financial affairs. Her admittance was made under the advice of a physician, and she was told that her stay in the home would be temporary (many patients are told this when they are admitted). Her physical condition was such that she needed 24-hour observation and care. She was incontinent at times, had badly swollen legs, and was confined to a wheelchair.

After five or six months in the facility, Mrs. Jones decided that she would like to leave and go back to her own apartment where she could live as she pleased. I explained to her that, although she had the right to leave the home, her doctor and her son would have to approve the new living arrangements because they were responsible for her safety. She would not accept this explanation because she knew that her physician would not recommend her release. At this point she was actually being held against her will.

Mrs. Jones became very adamant about returning to her apartment. She phoned friends, clergymen, her doctor, and even lawyers, seeking assistance and eventual release. Still, she could not find anyone to listen to her and cooperate with her efforts to return to society.

One day Mrs. Jones came into my office and told me she wanted to see an undertaker she knew and make arrangements for her burial. I contacted the funeral home and summoned the director, who came the next day to discuss plans for her internment. She insisted that he send her a lawyer so the plan could be put in legal form. The attorney was a warm and sympathetic man, and Mrs. Jones found herself telling him of her determination to get out of the facility. He agreed to help her. She had finally found someone who would listen, respect her intelligence, and insist that arrangements be finalized to permit her to return to her apartment.

Several days later Mrs. Jones sent a message to me by a nurse informing me that she would be leaving within the hour. A taxi soon arrived in front of the home and the driver came into the main office looking for Mrs. Jones to take her to her residence. I phoned the nurse in charge and requested that Mrs. Jones and all her belongings be brought to the main entrance. Then, in a matter of minutes, she was helped down the stairs, wheelchair and all, and into the cab. With her chin up and shoulders back, Mrs. Jones happily rode away. Her escape had been effected.

I thought at the time I would never see this lady again. However, one Saturday morning six weeks later, I parked my car in the parking lot of a busy shopping center and was walking toward the store when I heard a horn blowing frantically. I turned around and, to my astonishment, there was Mrs. Jones, *alone* at the wheel of a car, waving and smiling and shouting enthusiastically, "Hi, Mr. Bennett," as she drove confidently among the parked automobiles. How she had managed to get well enough to leave the wheelchair I never found out, but I was thrilled to see her and thought, "Good for her—I hope I have as much spunk if I'm ever taken to a nursing home." She was truly to be admired for such a remarkable accomplishment.

During my study, I was conscious of the physical configurations of traditional nursing homes and analyzed how they might affect the patients' capacity for exercising their drive for independence. Multi-floor facilities, I deduced, drastically limit this potential. Built because construction costs are less per square foot of space than for single-floor facilities, they incorporate inhibiting devices such as elevators and heavy fire doors at the bottoms of stairwells. These amenities are distinct barriers for many, particularly the handicapped, who wish to move about the institution or go out of doors.

The elevator is a fearful device for many patients. They become apprehensive when it travels between floors and wonder if it will stop at the right place. Some residents get feelings of claustrophobia when confined in such a close space. Because the nursing personnel are aware of these psychological difficulties, and for safety reasons (there is always the possibility that someone will push the wrong stop button and the car will get stuck between floors), most of the time patients have to have a staff escort when going from one floor to another. Frequently, the passengers have to order their "travel reservations" in advance, and must wait for the moment when a member of the staff is free to be their travel companion. Thus, elevators limit patients' freedom and independence considerably. I have observed many who stay in their wards for days at a time rather than go through the complicated procedure associated with the use of this mechanism.

Certain physical hazards are connected with the use of elevators. Patients can become trapped or injured by them in several ways. They have heavy automatic doors which close with substantial force. Many of the passengers are feeble and use canes, walkers, and other aids. Should these be in the way of a closing door (which sometimes happens), the patient can be knocked down and sustain injuries.

Several years ago some elderly people got trapped on an elevator in a home I was administering. One Sunday afternoon, as I was having dinner at home with my family, I received a phone call from a nurse who said, "The elevator is stuck, and I think someone is on it!" Naturally, the thought of an older person locked in an elevator was quite alarming. Like many homes, we did not have a formal, practiced procedure for handling an emergency of this kind.   I immediately phoned the fire department and the elevator company for assistance and rushed to the facility.

As I approached the closed first-floor elevator doors, I asked a group of nurses standing there who they thought might be trapped. They did not know but said that other staff members were checking all the beds and the signout book to try to determine who it could be. Then I asked everyone to be silent and called out into the closed doors, "Hello!" A faint voice, sounding like an echo coming from the distant end of a mile-long pipe, answered back, "Hello!" Simultaneously, a nurse who had checked our patient roster reported two or three of our guests missing. Sure enough, one or more of our charges were trapped between floors. Then I repeatedly called out, "Pull out the red emergency button! Pull Hard!"

By now 45 minutes had passed since I had received the emergency phone call. Suddenly a clicking sound came from the elevator shaft and the car started moving. It stopped in front of us and the doors opened. Inside were three women patients, all in their eighties. As suspected, one of them had pushed the emergency stop button while the car was in motion and there was no sound alarm to tell us what had happened (a situation soon corrected). They were all shaking and weak from fright. One was near a state of collapse. Naturally, the nursing staff was also unnerved—they had never had an experience of that kind. Following this frightening event, the staff appealed to me to enforce more vigorously the policy limiting patients' elevator travel without an escort. I complied and thereby further limited the freedom and independence of many of the residents.

Another reason why elevators restrict the movement of patients is that they contribute toward their sense of disorientation. I experienced this phenomenon while living in the nursing home—it was difficult for me to get oriented to my location within the building. The elevator seemed to compound this strange feeling. When traveling on it, I was not always sure which floor it would stop at. When the movement stopped and the doors opened, I was not absolutely certain I was at the desired destination. Floor numbers and colorful decor on the corridor walls were not completely orienting to me. When stepping off the elevator, I would glance up and down the corridor for some object or staff member I recognized to be sure I had arrived at the right place. Most always, it was the sight of a nurse whom I knew was assigned to my unit that told me where I was.

Comments from other patients being transported between floors along with me confirmed the idea that elevators restrict patients' freedom. They always appeared to feel apprehensive during the ride. I heard elderly people asking, "Where are we going?" "Is it moving?" and, "What floor are we on?" Invariably, when the car stopped and the doors opened, someone would say, "Is this the right place?" They always seemed to be a little confused.

Floor composition and covering was another element I considered during my analysis of the physical aspects of the nursing home environment. Until I was a patient, I believed it might be a good idea to use colorful carpeting in certain sections of homes to improve the esthetics of the interiors and to make the general atmosphere more homelike. This idea came from the journals and promotional material I had read depicting what a so-called modern nursing home should be. Certainly, it enriches the appearance of the interior and is impressive for visitors coming into the facility. Little thought may have been given, however, to the effect carpeting has on the movement of patients.

I found carpeting to be a barrier which obstructs the travel of people who use wheelchairs. It is much easier to roll this vehicle over other materials such as linoleum or hard tile floors. Carpet mouldings at entrances and doorways, I learned, present severe blockades. Many weakened patients simply do not have the strength to pass their wheelchairs over this elevated edging. I've seen people lean their bodies forward and rock back and forth rhythmically (as one rocks a car out of a snow bank) so they could gain momentum and make the chair move forward. Often they could not move past the obstruction at all and had to seek assistance from an able patient or a member of the staff.

Surprisingly, the nursing home operating regulations permit the use of carpeting in all patient areas. Only so-called "wet areas," such as laundries, bathrooms, utility rooms, and kitchens are excluded. Although bedrooms seldom have this kind of floor covering, it is frequently used in lounges, libraries, and general purpose areas. The regulatory standards, therefore, sponsor definite freedom barriers and hardships. Incontinent people are particularly deprived because administrators of some facilities disallow the use of carpeted areas by incontinent individuals. Some administrators also discourage wheelchair patients from entering these sections because they are concerned that the carpets will be spoiled by tire marks.

I remember a lady who was transferred to a facility I administered from an "exclusive" home in a nearby city. She pleaded with me not to let her go back there because they would not allow her to take her wheelchair into parts of the institution that had wall-to-wall carpeting. This limited her independence and made her feel discriminated against. Health regulations and standards, I now believe, should guarantee that all patients, incontinent or not, may use carpeted areas. If incontinency or tire marks are problems, the carpeting should be removed.

Respecting the Patients' Right to Make Decisions

Among the needs which the people living in the facilities I administered considered very important was the opportunity to make decisions. It became a significant part of my research and I sought the answer to the question, "Do patients have the chance to decide for themselves things which affect their daily lives?" I am sure most administrators would claim that their guests are given substantial decision making powers. This was my understanding, also, because I believed that most nurses are solicitous and allow the people they care for to have choice options. It is a mode covered in inservice training programs so the patients will be respected and treated as individuals. Now,

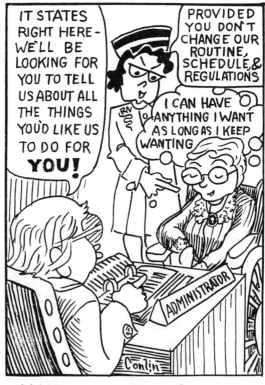

MAKING DECISIONS....

after having lived in a home for ten days, and after reflecting on my administrative experience, I realize that this opinion was not realistic. The opportunities for patients to make meaningful decisions are scarce.

Many influences existing in the traditional nursing home environment deny patients the opportunity to decide things for themselves. Established care systems and routines emulating the hospital environment are inflexible. As in hospitals, time schedules determine the hour residents arise in the morning, the time they dress, the time they eat, the time they participate in recreational activity programs, and the time they go to bed.

Nurses and aides do, however, try their best to respond to reasonable requests and they are usually as accommodating as they can possibly be. They may be seen pushing patients to and from their rooms and occasionally asking them if they want to satisfy an unmet need. Unfortunately, what they do for one they cannot always do for all. They work under pressures that make responding to every individual's wants an unrealistic expectation. There simply are not enough nurses and aides on duty to meet that kind of demand. Consequently, the care and personal service delivered is, by necessity, structured, and patients have no real opportunity to decide how it is to be carried out.

It is typical that when elderly people are admitted to a home they have played no part in formulating the plans for their new living arrangements. Out of respect, they may have been told about them, but they have not been seriously consulted. They receive information that is designed to induce them to *submit* to the move. Admissions into a nursing home are usually made from an acute care facility where the preliminary details are handled between a family member and the social service department of that institution. The will of the subject involved is not always a consideration. I have had numerous phone conversations with hospital social service personnel who were looking for a bed for one of their patients who was unaware of the arrangements being made. Sometimes, fortunately infrequently, the process of getting an older person into a home includes a family-concocted scheme, hoax, or trick, to misguide the patient and make it less traumatic for the person handling the affair. I have listened to many untruthful comments made to older men and women being admitted to the homes I administered. "It is only going to be for a little while," is quite popular. Other misleading statements that I've heard are, "Doctor wants you to come here where you'll get better care," and, "Just as soon as you get better we will bring you home." One of the most deceitful explanations I overheard was, "You'll only be here until we fix up your apartment, get you some clothes, and arrange for someone to take care of you." Most of the time, however, the newly admitted elderly person knows instinctively that he has been duped and is being deposited in the institution for the rest of his days.

The saddest admittance I ever witnessed involved an 80-year-old gentleman, Mr. Blue, who was brought into the nursing home by his son. In this case, the son had been completely honest with his dad but he could not get him to consent to being admitted to the home. I was aware, from previous conversations with members of the family, that the elderly man had become very forgetful and was wandering about during the night. Having this kind of a disability was a hazard to him and he needed 24-hour observation and care. As is often the case, this poor soul did not recognize the seriousness of his problem and wanted desperately to remain alone in his own home.

Mr. Blue was a refined and stately gentleman who had been professionally successful and affluent. Just being inside of a nursing home seemed to take him out of character. His son was very kind and tried his best to be open and honest as he explained to his father why it was necessary for him to have protection and medical care. Yet his dad would not give a signal of acceptance or approval to being placed in an institution. As I sat with them, I tried to lighten the trauma by being diplomatic and explaining the good attributes of nursing home life along with the rules families and patients are expected to obey. When I finished, Mr. Blue turned to his son, looked directly into his eyes, and said, "I never thought a son of mine would do this to me!" The remark hurt the son deeply; he choked, swallowed, and began to cry. There was nothing anyone could say to overcome the heartbreaking circumstance that was taking place. It was clear that Mr. Blue was facing the most depressing phase of his life. The tension was broken, however, when a nurse arrived and compassionately offered to escort our new guest to his bed. As I watched father and son walk in silence through the lounge doorway, headed toward Mr. Blue's room, I could not help thinking how sad and difficult it is for both patients and their families when nursing home care is needed.

I have become impressed by the fact that patients eventually accept the loss of their decision-making powers—that they become conditioned to the environment with its perpetual and boring routines, and ultimately adopt a stereotypical lifestyle. Allowing others to make decisions for them becomes a way of life. It occurred to me that it is this situation that some exponents of long term care theory allude to when speaking of "patient adjustment." Administrators and other nursing home personnel use these words when family members ask about their loved ones, or when inquiries are made from others seeking to know how admitted persons are finding institutional life. Such statements as, "Mr. Smith is adjusting well," or, "Mrs. Jones is not adjusting well," are phrases commonly used. What these responses really mean is that the person has or has not been discouraged from trying to make decisions; does or does not complain; or does or does not make demands of the staff. Those who insist upon having their share of attention are thought to be maladjusted. Having witnessed patients' withdrawal from decision-making situations, I have come to understand that the term "adjustment" is erroneous and inappropriate to use when describing the behavior of nursing home patients. They do not adjust—they *conform*. They do so by abdicating their need to exercise independence and allowing almost all of their decisions to be made for them.

Choice of Food—Serving Food Patients Like

The topic of conversation that comes up among patients most often in nursing homes is food. Mealtime is the major diversionary activity patients can look forward to every single day. What is to be served, or has been served, is always of special concern. Good or not so good, it undergoes critique and analysis by everyone in the facility. When individuals greet each other following a meal, the conversations usually start with the question, "How did you like that?" In-groups assemble to discuss their impressions about the kind, quantity, and quality of what they had just eaten. If the meals are found to be good, the morale of the whole institution will be elevated. If, on

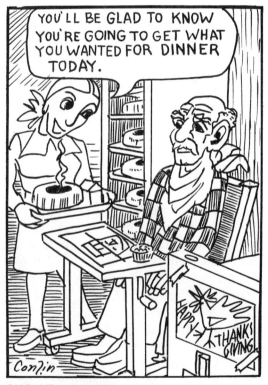

CHOICE OF FOOD . . . .

the other hand, the meals are found to be unsatisfactory, the morale of the whole facility will be lowered. In fact, negative reports seem to have a depressing effect on everyone, even the staff. Breakfast is the meal that receives the fewest condemnations. For all of these reasons, I believe that serving appetizing and nutritious meals is the biggest morale-building activity that can take place in nursing homes. It also improves the facility's image in the minds of people in the community.

When family members and others visit patients, they always bring up the subject of food. They continually inquire about the kinds of meals that are being served and want to know if their loved ones enjoy them. If they are told that the food is good, they are favorably impressed because it indicates that the patients are content and satisfied with the service they are receiving. It is also a method of measuring, to some degree, the quality of the patients' care.

Whether or not the patients have seen a menu in advance, they seem to know what is about to be served. They can tell by the time of day and the day of the week. They discuss the kinds of dishes that have been scheduled in the past and know when they will be repeated. The identity of the cook on duty at a given time signals in advance the kind and quality of upcoming meals.

It is not being implied that patients would not like to have options and be able to select what they eat, but they consider this an unrealistic expectation. My experience tells me that they would, indeed, enjoy choosing the style or kinds of meals they receive. Some people who were accustomed to certain ethnic dishes never see them again once they are admitted to a home. While a patient, I observed my colleagues having discussions about their favorite foods and how they wished they could have them again. I recall asking a patient, following a Friday dinner, how he had liked the meal. He said to me, "It was good, but I'll never get used to the food they serve here—it's not like I used to get at home." Upon being asked to be more specific, he responded in a resigned manner, "I'd have more fish—with mushrooms. But, you have to take what they give you—if you don't, you don't eat!'' When I recommended that he submit requests to the staff for special dishes he would like to have, he laughingly walked away, saying, ''Boy, are you senile! Why don't *you* try that? They'd think you had a lot of space between your ears!''

It was quite apparent that the nursing staff of the home where I stayed did everything they could to accommodate the patients and treat them like individuals. They were conscious of the many difficult problems connected with serving food and aware that some of their patients desired special kinds of dishes. When a dish was on the menu that they knew a particular person liked, they would inform the patient beforehand. One morning, I overheard a nurse say to one of the ladies, ''You're going to have your favorite dinner today!'' It was this staff member's way of telling her charge that the home did try to please the patients whenever it could. It sounded like an ordinary remark, but I'm sure it brightened that elderly lady's day.

The Need for Friends

Of all the basic human needs that I studied, it is the need of patients to have friends to which I had previously given the least amount of attention and forethought. As already mentioned, the traditional nursing home presents a hostile environment and does little to encourage visits from old acquaintances. As in the case of families, the opportunity for them to have intimate conversations is inhibited because of the lack of meaningful visiting space. Frequent encounters with disoriented and disturbed people and the depressing atmosphere discourages long and repetitive visits from friends.

Patients do, however, manage to compensate to some degree for the disassociation from people they knew in the past by adopting new friends from within the facility. Some have a favorite colleague whom they take into their confidence and with whom they

spend most of their socializing time. Cliques and in-groups
develop. They talk about things they did in the past, people they
used to know, and about experiences they once had. Not surprisingly, these in-groups become "reporting stations" for the
gossip and information of the day, which is then transmitted to
the rest of the population of the facility. I became a member of
one of these gatherings and spent many hours discussing things
that were happening in the home and listening to stories about
other patients and their past histories. It was here that I was able
to gather much of the information that enabled me to improve
my perspectives about the inner workings of nursing homes.

When thinking about the "friend need," I recalled a

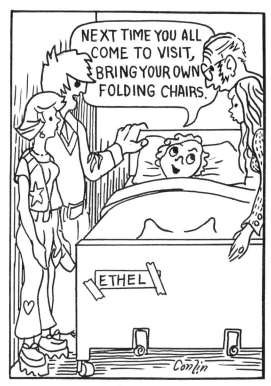

FAMILY AND FRIENDS....

patient who had been a guest in a facility I headed. He was about 85 years old and had been institutionalized for several years. He had had a successful professional career and had retired from a very responsible position in the community. This man had found it extremely difficult to adjust (conform) to nursing home life. His old friends, including outstanding members of the community with whom he had many years of friendship, did not come to see him. On a number of occasions he complained that he could not find anyone in the home to converse with because "They don't have anything in common with me." Understandably, his interests and past involvements in the professional world removed him from most of the other patients, who had had different experiences and lifestyles. Consequently, he was very unhappy and displeased at having to live in a nursing home.

I realize now that special measures need to be employed in homes to assist patients to maintain old relationships and make new ones. The staff can help with the task of keeping them in touch with people they knew before they were admitted. In addition, bed assignments should not be based solely on physical-medical conditions or where a vacancy happens to fall. Neither should the ability of a patient to pay be the determinant of where he or she lives. Certainly, if the facility had met its responsibility to the man just described by deviating from standard ways to help him cope with his predicament, his final years could have been made more peaceful. This particular experience taught me that the higher people go socially, educationally, and economically, the farther they tumble, meaning the harder it is for them to accept nursing home life.

One might think that multi-bed rooms serve the purpose of stimulating friendships and increasing social interaction among patients. This is not true. It is my experience that the opposite takes place. Patients do not automatically become intimately friendly with those living in their room. It is usual, in fact, for them to fall into conflict with one another. This happens because of disagreements over space use, displeasure over the activities of roommates, excessive noise, disturbances during the night, and many other factors, including manipulation of the privacy curtains, windows, and window shades. As a patient, at times I found myself feeling somewhat anti-social over my roommate's use of the divider screen. I didn't like being closeted in at night or being denied sunlight during the day. I frequently left the room to seek conversations with other people who had more in common with me. It is ordinary to see patients sitting next to their beds in silence, some with their heads down, making it quite obvious they do not wish to be bothered by the individuals who have been placed near them. Real sociability and friendships are cultivated outside of patients' rooms where acquaintances can be selected on the basis of mutual interests.

The small size of patients' rooms, and the kind of furniture used in them, do little to accommodate visitors. The regulations do not require more than one easy chair per bed. This is hardly enough to induce visitors (families in particular) to stay by the patient's side for any length of time. If more than one person visits, there is no place for them to sit down.

Choosing What to Wear

One indication of the quality of the services delivered in a home is how the patients are dressed. If the residents have a daily change of outer clothing, if their garments are pressed, and if they look neat and clean, it is a fair assumption that an effort is being made to improve their well-being. This is a sign that the staff is functioning at maximum level and, in all probability, that the personnel assignments exceed the state-sponsored minimum quotas. If, however, residents' clothing looks unkempt, or some patients seem to wear the same dress over and over again, or many patients unnecessarily wear the standard nursing home uniform (the ''johnny''), it is reasonable to believe that an updating of the service is in order. The latter description, unfortunately, typifies the appearance of some people living in traditional geriatric environments. It is a byproduct of: 1) the many complications associated with the dressing problem, and 2) the failure of applied systems to provide adequate supervision, employee training, and numbers of staff personnel.

Laundering patients' clothes is a tremendous obstacle for many nursing homes. Frequently they do not have efficient facilities or equipment. It is ordinary for many homes to have the laundry done by commercial companies which specialize in serving institutions. Pressing garments is an extra effort and an extra cost, and financial restraints cause some homes to forgo this amenity. Clothes get washed frequently—over and

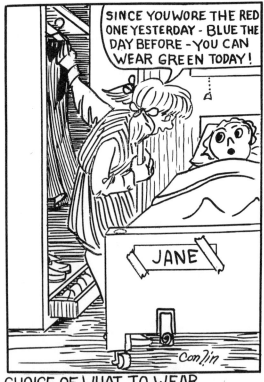

CHOICE OF WHAT TO WEAR. . . .

over again—but the repetitive washing takes the texture out of the materials and, when dry, they sometimes become incendiary—a hazard for smoking patients. Excessive laundering also causes clothing to become torn and lose color. Families should remove their patients' old garments, and replace them with new ones as often as possible. This will go a long way in helping the facility overcome some of the problems associated with dressing patients. Unfortunately, some families fail to provide their relatives with adequate changes of dress, which makes it necessary for the staff of the home to provide secondhand substitutes.

Just keeping track of which clothes belong to which patients is difficult. Identification markings applied to the garments eventually get washed off, with the result that clothes are frequently found hanging in the wrong person's closet. Complicating all this are the many incontinent patients who require many changes of dress each day.

With respect to patients having a choice of what they wear, the reality is that this option is often removed. During the early morning hours when dressing normally occurs, the staff is rushing to meet strict time schedules. Some nurses and aides are attentive; others are not. Quite frequently, it is a case of a staff member reaching in the clothes closet, taking out a garment, and saying to the patient, "How would you like to wear this today?" Knowing that the staff is busy, and thinking a rejection would indicate a lack of cooperation, the patient says, "Fine." Actually, the problem is so involved for patients who wish to be dressed neatly, that many lose interest and just accept what they are handed.

I had an interesting dress problem experience involving a patient named Miss Gray. It demonstrates how patients can react when they are deprived of suitable clothing. Miss Gray had had a stroke and was paralyzed on the right side. She couldn't walk and had impaired speech. Because of unusual welfare difficulties, she received a meager subsistence allowance for her personal needs and was unable to purchase clothes or even treats.

She had to wear old and unattractive dresses and was always agitated, heartsick, and depressed. This condition persisted until the director of nurses and the activities director took a special interest in her welfare. Due to their urgings and tenacity, the personal needs subsistence allowance was increased, clothes were brought into the home for Miss Gray to purchase and wear, and there was even extra money for her to enjoy miscellaneous treats. A dramatic change soon took place. She didn't get agitated very much anymore; she smiled frequently; became content; and was proud to wear decent new clothes again. Thanks to my two astute staff members, her dignity was restored.

Patients' Religious Needs

When I began the basic human need study discussed in Chapter 3, I hypothesized that religion would show up as one of the highest in priority needs. This was expected because I believed that older people, being concerned about their health, were preoccupied with the hereafter and focused their thoughts on religion. The averaged-out ratings of the participants in the experiment, however, placed religion tenth in order of importance. This was a surprise, and it caused me to be very conscious of the religious factor during the period of time when I was a patient.

The facility I was admitted to had all the major western faiths represented among the patient population. I did not know the exact percentage of patients per denomination, but I judged it was about evenly distributed. A large room in the home was set aside for use as a chapel on weekends and clergymen visited the patients regularly. With this kind of religious orientation, I expected an outstanding display of peoples' interest in their faith and, quite possibly, an indication that part of my research was fallible.

To gain a greater understanding about how patients think about their religious needs, I went to church with them on Sunday. Those who were there were happy and grateful to have a chance to deviate from the regular daily routine, and a lot of socializing was going on in the room. I overheard several comments about how fortunate they were to have chaplains who visited them each week. But not many people were there. Out of a population of over 150, only 12, including myself, were in the room. This did not seem to represent much enthusiasm on the part of the patients to attend church. I was so surprised by the low number of participants that I wondered if everyone who would have liked to be there was aware that the rites were being held.

Comparing this experience with church attendance in a home I administered is even more interesting. This institution had a formal chapel and employed Catholic and Protestant chaplains. Mass and church services were conducted every Sun-

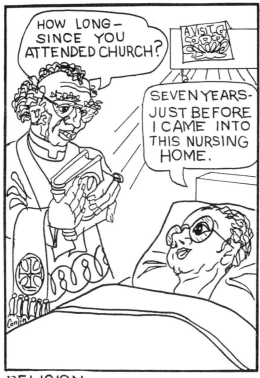

RELIGION . . . .

day and on all the other special holy days. Seventy-five percent of the patients were Catholic, and the balance were Protestant, with two being Jewish. An average of approximately 45 out of a population of 134 patients attended the regular weekly church services. Although this certainly represents a greater response than that demonstrated in the home where I stayed, it makes the reason why these same people failed to show religion high in priority even more puzzling.

After thinking about this question and discussing it with members of my staff, I came to the conclusion that attending church in a nursing home cannot substitute for the real experience of going to church in the community. Once in a home, association with the religious ritual as it was previously known becomes lost. Faith then emerges as an individual expression to be satisfied in individual ways. This is evident when you see patients reading the Bible or saying rosary while seated by their bedsides, in lounges, and in corridors of the facility.

Chapels and chaplains do not, by themselves, fully satisfy patients who are devout and have been loyal members of a congregation or parish. Alone, they do little to maintain continuity between individuals and their former religious experiences. When older people go into a nursing home they are removed from the kind of worship and ritual they formerly enjoyed. The chapel is not the "real church" they were familiar with for many years. Most importantly, no one can substitute for the priest, minister, or rabbi they used to see and hear each Sabbath.

Ever since I became a nursing home administrator, I've attended numerous seminars and other educational programs that stressed the importance of recognizing the religious needs of patients. I've been taught that this is a basic responsibility of administrators and that lists of the residents' former parishes, churches, temples, and clergymen should be kept and maintained. Pastoral care programs, making provisions for special days of worship, and contacting preachers in times of crisis, are ways suggested to accomplish spiritual goals. Obviously, these measures are important and should be normal operating functions in nursing homes, but by no means should these efforts mean that homes have a basic responsibility to satisfy the religious needs of all the patients. The institution cannot do this alone. *The community and all the churches in the community have this responsibility.* Administrators need to be concerned with the question, "What is the community doing to help satisfy the patients' needs for religion, and why can't church representatives come to the nursing home each Sabbath and take patients, wheelchairs and all, into society where they may see old friends and attend mass or services in their former houses of worship?" Certainly, many parishes and congregations must have worshippers who will practice their faith and provide a vehicle and the energy to make this possible. It is something that can be done and should be done, especially when the patients have contributed financially and given other support to their churches over the years.

Patients' Financial Affairs

One of the most devastating experiences that a nursing home patient can have is losing control over his own financial affairs. This is initiated before admittance, and usually after the patient has been through a long period of illness and hospitalization. When the person can no longer be kept in a hospital or at home, someone, most often a family member, takes over the responsibility of arranging for continued care. This representative, in consort with a hospital or other agency such as a welfare office, will complete the financial details, contact a nursing home, and reserve a bed. The patient, at this point, seldom knows what is happening. He rarely knows what the cost of the institutional care is or what the other related expenses are. Actually, the patient is too stressed to comprehend clearly the plan that has been formulated for him.

There are two general categories of people who enter homes—private paying persons and those on public assistance.

In the latter category, the cost of care will be paid by sponsoring public assistance agencies. Most patients in long term care facilities are welfare supported.

The facility does not have information about the personal financial affairs of private paying patients. The families have this knowledge and it is their responsibility to keep loved ones informed of expenditure obligations or arrangements which are made in their behalf. The facility can only present statements to these residents that show what the costs have been.

As for public assistance cases, it is the responsibility of the sponsoring agency's representatives to ensure that the financial details are explained to their clients. They have all the background financial and eligibility data on the people in nursing homes under their auspices. Unfortunately, some social workers for sponsoring agencies seldom visit patients for that purpose. This was true in the facilities I administered. The welfare social worker visited the institution mainly to have his clients' annual recertification documents filled out. He would hand a large quantity of them to the director of nurses to prepare for him. He had too many patients to serve, too little time to explain the details to each one, and wouldn't complete the forms himself.

Most nursing homes do keep their patients informed about per diem charges made against them by the facility, as required by a federally mandated Patients' Bill of Rights. They do so by issuing accounting reports (usually quarterly). In addition, social service personnel are available to explain the charges when necessary. This does not mean, however, that the patients' opinions are being solicited about the expenses indicated on these statements. The purpose of the notices is merely to tell people what the costs have been over a given period of time. In other words, this particular document pertains mostly to transactions which have occurred after the fact. As indicated earlier, since the facilities do not have the complete financial history of the patients, it is the obligation of families and third party payers to give the patients a voice in their economic affairs.

Patients sponsored by public assistance agencies receive a monthly subsistance allowance. This is to enable them to buy clothes, toilet items, treats, and miscellaneous items. The amount of this subsidy in Massachusetts is $35 at the present time. Supervision over this spending money may be handled in one of three ways: 1) It may be given directly to the patients, 2) it may be put in the charge of family members, or 3) it may be under the supervision of the facility. The latter alternative is used when there are no responsible family members to take charge of the patient's personal affairs. Only the very alert and able people handle their own funds. The others have had this responsibility removed from them.

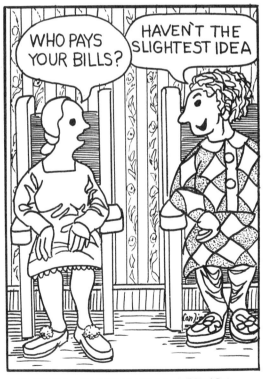

CONTROL OF FINANCIAL AFFAIRS . . .

Although most families use the subsistance money prudently, and have the interest of their relatives at heart, a few do not, and there have been instances where family members have spent this money on themselves. Heavy-drinking or debt-ridden next of kin find it very useful. Sometimes they deposit it, under the name of another person, in a bank. On occasion I have petitioned the Social Security Office to appoint me as a patient's Representative Payee so I could intercept this allowance, place it under the control of the nursing home, and eliminate abuses. Not only are some patients being deprived by the current methods of handling subsistance allowances, but millions of federal dollars are being misappropriated in the process. Yet it is a problem that can easily be corrected.

When the money is held by the nursing home, it often accumulates because it may be difficult to spend. Since the facility satisfies all of the patients' life-sustaining needs, if a patient does not smoke, does not eat treats, and postpones the purchase of clothes, this cash goes unspent.

The magnitude of this situation is greater when considering what happens to the patients' funds when patients die. There is always a surplus of cash left when that happens. Homes that control the allowances may return them to the sponsoring agency (a requirement in Massachusetts). When a fund is under the supervision of family members or, as occasionally happens, of the patients themselves, it either gets spent or stays in the bank. Unfortunately, state agencies are so burdened and so understaffed that they cannot effectively monitor the dispensing of all their clients' funds.

To expect that all nursing home patients should have control over their financial affairs is unrealistic. Many are not able to handle them. Some cannot write, speak, or think clearly. Most recognize their limitations and prefer to have family members keep their records and pay their bills for them. Therefore, it is mainly the very alert and independence-seeking people who are deprived of the financial control need.

It is not being implied that all residents of homes are un-
concerned about their business matters. They may have ab-
dicated their responsibility for them, but many are interested
in knowing how their affairs are being handled. As an administrator, I've been asked by numerous patients if their
board and room is being paid, how it is being paid, and who
pays it for them. Over the years I've played the role of a welfare
department social worker in explaining payment mechanisms and
benefits to residents. Sometimes patients are suspicious that
their personal affairs are being mishandled. I recall the case of
a patient who came into my office upset and in tears, worrying
that her sister was arranging through legal means to take control
of her bank accounts. In the course of our conversation she
said to me, "I love my sister and she loves me, but I'm afraid
she also loves my money—she wants to be able to spend my savings
without asking me." When I spoke to the sister a few days later,
I learned that there was no intention on her part to violate the
wishes of her complaining sister. It was a situation where the
lady paying the bills wanted, for convenience, to do so without
having to bring checks for her sister's signature and bills and
bankbooks into the facility.

Patients' Need to Communicate with the Outside

The complications involved in communicating with friends and
relatives tend to separate nursing home patients from the community. For those who wish to write letters, even getting a
postage stamp can be a difficult logistical problem. In addition, some residents have poor eyesight, coordination
disabilities, paralysis of the fingers and hands, and require
assistance with writing and reading letters. For similar reasons,
some people cannot easily make telephone calls. There are not
enough nurses and aides on duty to respond to the residents'
personal social requests all the time. Most always, special
demands have to wait for a moment when the staff is not busy, but

requests made in advance frequently get forgotten. Many patients hesitate to ask staff members to help them write letters and make phone calls because they fear such requests will be regarded as impositions. They finally lose interest in satisfying their communication needs and simply don't bother to upset the nurses' routines.

As I sat in my wheelchair in the lounge one evening, this problem was acted out for me. I overheard the conversation of two elderly ladies, Mrs. Black and Mrs. White, who were seated nearby. Mrs. Black had been asked to contact her sister by phone that day. Because she was wheelchair-bound and had arthritic hands, she was unable to use the phone alone. Mrs.White, knowing about the need of her friend to use a telephone, was in-

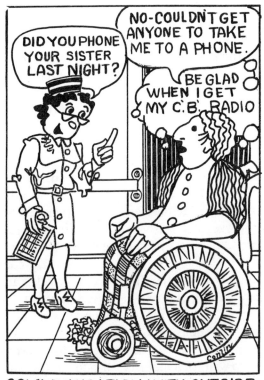

COMMUNICATION WITH OUTSIDE..

sisting that the call be made. When Mrs. Black said she would like to make the call but didn't have the necessary change, Mrs. White obligingly offered to give it to her. But Mrs. Black, with a tone of resignation in her voice, answered, "Oh, no. I can't call now—the nurses are too busy. I'll call tomorrow."

I did not know whether that telephone call was important, but it seemed to me that the systems operating in the home should have been flexible enough to allow Mrs. Black to use the phone regardless of the time of day. Certainly, I thought, this must happen often and there must be many others who impose this deprivation upon themselves and pass up the pleasure of talking to a friend or relative.

Significantly, there are no meaningful regulations pertaining to the use of telephones in nursing homes. One public phone for the use of 30 to 130 patients may be considered sufficient. Coin operated phones are relied upon for contact with people living in the community, and the use of free phones is not mandated. Unfortunately, not all patients have the physical capacity (or, frequently, the change) to make calls. Those with crippled hands, poor eyesight, and those who need help to ambulate are deprived of making calls almost entirely. As in the case of satisfying other social needs, the limited staff makes it complicated for them to get assistance.

It is unfair to imply that the personnel in homes never give a hand to people who want to use the telephone. Most are willing to give this aid whenever they can find time outside of pressing duties. Sometimes they will allow people, particularly the severely handicapped, to use the free business units in the medical office. The fact of the matter is, however, that too many of the patients have this need and that there are too few nurses, aides, and phones to distribute unlimited telephone use equitably among the total population of the facility.

Nursing home design specifications fail to make recommendations relative to the placement of telephones. Few facilities have installed connection jacks next to the beds for those who are able to use them and can afford to pay the charges.

Most frequently, the instrument is located in an open alcove or in a corridor where conversations are within hearing distance of passing visitors, staff members, and others. Some patients I knew always waited until night when most of their colleagues had retired before making their calls. They did this so they could maintain confidentiality and prevent personal affairs from becoming generally known around the home. Quite often, they made calls during staff mealtimes and evenings, when there were fewer staff members on duty, so they could speak in private and tell their families about affairs taking place in their units. They did not want to subject themselves to possible reprisals for expressing displeasure about their care.

That patients need to have unlimited access to telephones is something that the nursing home system evades. Eliminating and restricting the use of phones is a means of holding down operating expenses—a priority which seemingly must take precedence over the basic human need to communicate.

Not until I was a patient and studied the nursing home environment did I fully realize how much the communication need is deprived. I became aware that it is through conversations with people familiar to them—friends, relatives, and old acquaintances—that patients are able to remain connected with their community, loved ones, and former experiences. Disconnection from all this causes anxieties, disappointments, and sadness. I know this to be true because I had these feelings myself during a stage of my research. They were among the most disturbing feelings I ever had in my life (the episode referred to is the experience I had on my sixth night as a patient when an uncontrollable urge made me want to phone my wife and leave the facility). I had reached a breaking point and tears came into my eyes. I then found it inconceivable that older people, alert and feeling well, have to spend their remaining days in a traditional nursing home environment. Yet I had to admire their ability to cope with the most difficult aspects of living an institutional life—depression, fear, loneliness, and separation from the people they love. *Being able to talk over the telephone without logistical barriers is basic and vital.*

Realities of Patients' Needs for Recognition and Accomplishment

Although numerous interesting concepts came forth during the process of gathering material for this book, the matter of recognition emerged in a very special way. I became troubled over the fact that this need was considered by the patients as low in priority. It seemed to me that everyone has an intense need to be appreciated and respected. What is there about the nursing home environment, I wondered, which might cause people to lower their feelings of self-esteem and view this need as secondary? The depressing thought that they just don't care about themselves any more crossed my mind. Is it a fact, I asked myself, that the reality of their past contributions to society and their personal achievements have been stored away so deeply in their subconscious minds that nothing can restore their sense of pride? Sorrowfully, I came to the conclusion that this may be a valid assumption. Nursing homes that I know do not sponsor effective efforts to perpetuate service delivery modes which honor the needs for recognition and accomplishment.

The analysis of the recognition factor was done within the framework of Webster's definition, i. e., recognition means "identification of a person or thing as *being known* to one." I interpreted this to mean that, in order to acknowledge people in a true sense, one should show awareness and respect for *everything* known about them, including what they have done in the past. Simply complimenting people about their appearance, expressing pleasure over the recent accomplishment of some task, or extending greetings is only a small part of showing genuine appreciation for other persons. Unfortunately, nursing home patients' backgrounds are sometimes secreted for no reason other than that it has always been a medical mode to maintain strict confidentiality about patients' histories. As a result, many staff members, particularly nurses' aides and other operational level personnel, do not have the information that would enable them to give full recognition to the people they serve. In other words, more is involved than just making courteous statements when someone is to be recognized. Older people have a natural desire to be accepted in terms of their whole selves. Their past histories, former contributions, and attainments are all vital parts of the composite which makes them what they are at present.

There are other reasons why patients are deprived of recognition once they enter a nursing home. The denial of opportunities to satisfy all of the needs reviewed here contributes toward this. The loss of possessions and of decision-making powers, to mention just two, very definitely diminish a person's feelings of self-worth. In addition, the stereotyped environments, designed to treat everyone in a common manner, lessen the probability of preserving individuality. The feelings that such need-deprivations engender have been expressed to me on a number of occasions by patients who said, "When you get old, no one cares about you any more!"

The relevance of institutionalized people having an opportunity to experience accomplishments is something not fully appreciated by many of those working in nursing homes (including some administrators). Because our society is so youth oriented, people associate the desires to achieve and create with younger persons. Senior citizens, on the other hand, particularly those living in long term care facilities, are often thought of as being too old to be interested in being productive and as lacking in ambition. Consequently, many elderly individuals who possess social and other special skills go undetected, with no chance to use their capabilities. Skilled and creative people can be found among those who do little else but pass the time of day "waiting to be called." The reality is, however, that all alert and able people have unused talents, interests, and skills. Older people with disabilities but who feel well are no different than anyone else. It is natural for them to want to be creative and to set and conquer goals. As with younger people, it is the way they can maintain feelings of usefulness and self-worth. All employees of nursing homes should understand these dynamics and encourage the delivery of effective systems which seek out people with hidden talents and help them satisfy their innate needs for accomplishment.

Most nursing homes do try to help patients to be creative and productive to some extent. In fact, more is done in homes to satisfy their needs for accomplishment than is done for any of the other needs studied. (This is somewhat ironic in view of its being judged lowest in importance by the patients in our study.) It is the implementation of comprehensive recreational activity programs which accounts for this. These efforts make it possible for the residents to use their craft and social art skills by creating various objects and participating in group activities. Actually, if an equivalent amount of concern was demonstrated within the nursing home field, particularly by regulatory agencies, for satisfying all of the other patient needs, homes would have vastly improved living environments.

The Disassociation from Community Activities

Once people enter a nursing home they are separated from normal activities taking place in the community. They become isolated, with little hope for interaction or physical contact with friends and organizations on the outside. The reasons for this are threefold. First, they are generally considered incapable of community involvement; second, the community does not recognize a responsibility to continue its ties with them; and third, homes do not always have the resources to carry out meaningful efforts to make participation in society's affairs possible.

As mentioned in Chapter 6, more than half of the residents

are mentally alert and rational people. The idea that all patients are incapable of or disinterested in participating in community affairs is false. Many would enjoy shopping trips to town and attendance at the numerous social events taking place there. This is evident when they are seen looking out of the windows trying to get a glimpse at what is happening "out there." Many receive and read newspapers and magazines and listen to the radio and watch TV to keep updated on current events. The fact is, they demonstrate that they have the same interests they had when living in society. Their conversations include politics, sports, world events, and other topics associated with community life.

That the community does not recognize its responsibility toward nursing home patients is apparent when it is realized that community organizations seldom take people out of the facilities into society. For example, as already indicated, most churches do not provide transportation and escorts to make it possible for these incarcerated people to attend their in-town churches. An equivalent lack of concern is shown by other groups and organizations, such as civic clubs, commercial enterprises, cultural organizations, and labor and political groups. For some unexplained reason, this responsibility is considered as belonging solely to the nursing home rather than to society at large. The interest that *is* shown by the community usually comes during holiday seasons, when an abundance of charity is generally demonstrated.

This chapter has discussed the failure of the nursing home system to satisfy patients' basic human needs in numerous instances. It has also uncovered many complex and frustrating problems associated with the delivery of appropriate care. The next chapter is an overview of the system, wider in scope, which will give a better understanding of the traditional nursing home environment and will reveal more of the elements, inherent in the system, that foster patient deprivations.

8

Why Patient Deprivations Occur

In the 60s, when federal legislation made it possible to provide care for all of society's disabled elderly people, nursing homes accepted the task under most difficult circumstances. The sudden increase in a demand for beds, and the impromptu expansion of the number of institutions, presented obstacles that the health system had never faced before. Existing operational standards and guidelines failed to address the numerous new problems that were arising. The new long term facilities were built to conform to specifications originated for sophisticated hospitals rather than for *homes* and were later found to be incompatible with the real needs of most patients. An equitable payment mechanism for physicians which would encourage their consistant visits to residents was not established. Neither was an efficient monitoring system put in place so health agencies could guide developers through the expansion stage and ensure uniform and appropriate long term care. Actually, nursing homes needed a lengthy trial- and error-period to refine and perfect the service delivery procedures. Now, after having served elderly disabled people for 15 or more years, homes are sometimes held solely accountable for failures inherent in the system. In reality, however, most all of the malevolence attributed to them is directly related to regulatory restraints and care modes which were in place at the time that the need for long term care exploded.

This book has elaborated on many deprivations and hardships endured by patients in nursing homes. Yet, given the systems and operating standards which make them what they are, most are well run and provide a valuable service to society and the thousands of people they serve. They have provided an effective means of separating the specialty of long term care from high-cost acute care and have played a significant part in the effort to minimize overall health costs. In fact, nursing home service is the most reasonable component of health service available. For example, a typical daily rate of $45 reflects an hourly cost of just $1.88. This is remarkable considering that it includes 24-hour nursing service, housekeeping, meals, recreational programs, social service, and a multitude of other amenities. No other sector of the economy offers so much for so little.

Most of the publicized abuses and deficiencies associated with nursing home life fall in the categories of physical neglect and indifference. Among those that have received widescale publicity are incidents of failure to keep patients clean, serving unsatisfactory meals, excessive frequency of accidents, offensive odors, over-restraining patients, and insufficient nurse staffing. These revelations, however, are not indicative of the kind of care delivered in every facility. They represent accounts of isolated episodes. Unfortunately, they damage the reputation and image of every good nursing home.

This chapter will deal with the factors that cause patient injustices, and will offer concepts which, when put to work, will help to prevent them from happening.

A number of factors connected to the nursing home system foster most patient injustices. Some of these factors are government sponsored and some are historically derived. They are:

1. The effects of the federally supported certificate-of-need laws.
2. The absence of meaningful precedents for appropriate long term care.
3. A lack of awareness of patients' basic human needs among health care professionals.
4. Barriers existing between medically- and nonmedically-oriented disciplines.
5. The absence of meaningful sanitation standards.
6. The absence of pertinent educational programs for nursing home personnel.
7. Cost controls which limit necessary staffing.

The Effects of the Certificate-of-Need Laws

The regulations that are most influential in creating and perpetuating substandard and abusive practices in homes are the certificate-of-need laws. These acts, administered and enforced by regional and state public health agencies, control the number of nursing home beds. They limit the construction of new facilities and the expansion of existing ones by requiring developers to obtain permits. The number of beds allowed in a region is based on demographic formulas which anticipate the number of beds needed per thousand persons who are over 65. These formulas do not allow for a meaningful oversupply of beds and do not take into consideration the substandard care delivered by some existing facilities. The direct consequence of these regulations is that competition, based on quality of care, is eliminated among homes. Poorly operated homes are protected and preserved by the certificate-of-need laws. Many fine facilities that make sincere efforts to deliver good care have their reputations tarnished by a few unfit facilities shielded under these laws.

Absence of Meaningful Precedents for Appropriate Long Term Care

Another significant factor forming the basis for substandard care is the absence of an ideal nursing home model. This is not true of acute-care facilities. They operate under perfected guidelines, employ skilled health professionals who are trained in appropriate disciplines, and pursue standardized, cure-oriented goals. Patients throughout the country can expect to receive good care and service in these institutions. The quality of the long term care delivered in nursing homes, however, has not yet been perfected and made uniform. It varies among homes even when they are physically close to one another in the same community. The unique and special disciplines involved are still in the process of being defined, refined, and standardized so health agencies can monitor an expected quality of care.

Lack of Awareness of Patients' Basic Human Needs Among Health Care Professionals

The national effort, supported by health planners across the country, is directed toward impeding the growth of the nursing home system. Long term care in an institutional setting is regarded as a liability and as an inefficient means of serving older people. But, until such time as health care advances to a point where it can prevent the disabilities associated with old age, *something that will not happen,* the need for institutional care for older people will continue. This cold, hard fact is not taken seriously by influential health planners today. The thrust of their work appears to be toward the nebulous goal of eliminating the need for most nursing home care. As a result, only token efforts are being made to improve the environments and services of homes, and the elderly people living in them have been virtually abandoned under the pretexts that 1) their care costs are too high, and 2) that some time in the future most all disabled elders will be able to receive 24-hour care through community-based support programs. In the meantime, thousands of patients who are living in these facilities could benefit from innovative and improved standards of care. Instead, they are being made to forgo satisfying many of their needs and made to wait until substitute care measures come into being at some unspecified future date. Their rights are being traded off by health professionals who promote the idea that the needs of future old people are more important than the needs of disabled elders living in homes today.

In view of this, sponsors of homes are not receiving adequate support and encouragement to improve their environments and to continue their operations as respected components of the health system. This accounts for some of the deficiencies attributed to nursing homes. In spite of it all, however, thousands of older human beings are receiving good care in them.

A lack of awareness of the needs of elderly institutionalized people is shown in other ways. Homes can be built almost anywhere and they are sometimes found wedged between other buildings. There are no standards requiring that they have suitable outside grounds with walks, patios, trees, or picnic areas where patients can exercise and enjoy the outdoor scenery This aspect of nursing home development offers little in the way of incentive for patients to leave the inside environments.

One large nursing home with which I am familiar exemplifies how many needs can be unnecessarily sacrificed for monetary and material reasons. The board of directors of this particular facility had engaged the services of development specialists and an architect to enlarge their facility.

The development plan which was ultimately approved and sanctioned by state health officials called for the erection of a new 120-bed building and renovation of the existing home. However, rather than construct the new building first and then move the patients from the existing facility into it after it was completed, the two construction jobs were to be done *simultaneously.* The rationale for this was that the project would be completed sooner and that there would be certain construction cost savings. The deprivations and inconveniences which were bound to be the lot of the elderly people living in the older institution while it was being renovated were not thought to be significant enough to justify losing time and perhaps some money.

Major and total renovation of the nursing home commenced with many old and disabled people living in it. The magnitude of the harm, hardships, and disruptions that the patients endured was greater than anything I had ever known or heard of. Four-bed rooms were made to house six patients, and two-bed rooms were used to accommodate four. There was very little space between the beds; there were no clothes closets for those who over-occupied the rooms; the patients' recreational area was eliminated completely; and loud hammering noises and plaster dust permeated the entire environment.

The renovation work went on for over a year. As it proceeded, the patients were moved like "logs" from room to room, some as many as four or five times within a period of just a few months. Many of them became mentally confused, disturbed, and depressed. The physical condition of some regressed. Pressures on the nursing staff multiplied and the morale of the entire facility was at an all-time low. Even the patients' families were distressed and worried.

Fortunately, the renovation work was suspended to await completion of the new building halfway through the project. It was not suspended for patient hardship reasons, but because the contractor was having logistical difficulties. In other words, the patients were in his way. The cost savings turned out to be considerably less than the board of directors had been led to believe, and it became evident that the development scheme was wrong, ill-advised, and financially unsound.

Episodes of this kind do not become generally known. It is related here in the hope of discouraging such insensitive procedures from occurring again. In this particular case, there is no possible way to explain away such massive injustices when they could and should have been avoided.

Barriers Existing Between Medically- and Nonmedically-Oriented Disciplines

Professionals working in hospitals and nursing homes function according to a prescribed medical hierarchy. The physician ranks at the top and exercises the greatest amount of influence. His judgment is usually taken as supreme and infallible, and he can affect, usually without question, all of the care procedures and services employed to improve the well-being of patients. Next in order of influence come the other medical people—registered nurses, radiologists, laboratory technicians, dietitians, licensed practical nurses, nurses' aides, and so on, with nonmedically-oriented categories, such as social service personnel, recreational activity staff, houseworkers, kitchen workers, and others stationed at the bottom of the scale.

This order of influence is conducive to quality patient care in short term, acute care hospitals, where cure of illness and disease is the primary objective. The education and training of physicians and the other health professionals are in harmony with the ultimate goal—cure. It does not follow, however, that this traditional order of influence is conducive to quality care in nursing homes. The objectives and goals are different in this part of the health system. Cure is unlikely and has a secondary meaning. The basic objectives in homes involve not only the employment of medical procedures to maintain the patients' maximum physical wellness, but also measures to satisfy those human needs which enhance the attainment of a good quality of life. Physicians and other acute care health professionals have not, by tradition, been trained or motivated to focus on these aspects of care as primary goals. It is only recently that the reciprocal relationship between a person's psychological state and physical state has been taken seriously and recognized during the care process. The implementation of care modes which honor *all* of the patient's needs on an equal basis is vital in the delivery of nursing home care.

It is employees at the middle and lower part of the influence scale, those who have direct contact and close association with the patients, who know best if their basic human needs are being satisfied. They are more apt to know if families visit, if patients have the opportunity to go outside, if freedoms are being taken away, and so forth. Total care means filling patients' social, psychological, medical, and environmental needs, and its application depends on judgments and ideas that come from staff members on every level—from nurses' aides, houseworkers, kitchenworkers, and all the others. When their input is removed from the process of developing care plans and operating procedures, maximum service is not delivered and personnel conflicts develop.

An experience I had with an elderly married couple living in a facility I administered demonstrates how conflicts come about over medical and nonmedical modes. This couple had been confined to the nursing home for months. The husband had just recovered from a fractured hip and his wife had recovered from an abdominal operation. Both were ambulatory, alert, and responsible individuals.

One morning they visited me in my office and asked if they could take a taxi into town for a lobster dinner. I told them that this was their right but that, before going, they should inform the supervisor of nurses on duty at the time. A few minutes later the nurse came to me complaining forcefully about letting her patients leave the facility. She was afraid that the man might fall again and refracture his hip. It was not part of her rationale that it would be psychologically therapeutic for them to get out of the confining environment and enjoy a good meal in a nice restaurant. I had to insist that the couple be permitted to leave. They had their lobster dinner and returned to the home, hip intact. They were feeling much better when they came back than before they left. I thought at the time that they might even have indulged in a martini.

Interdisciplinary acceptance barriers (IABs), another byproduct of acute care which has been carried over to the nursing home environment, discourage intimate participation by the personnel in one category in the affairs of those of another. It results from the mode, necessarily practiced in hospitals, which respects and fosters the expertise of disciplinary skills and places heavy emphasis on the confidentiality of patients' affairs. This concept rightfully fixes responsibility within defined perimeters and advances the cause of developing departmental efficiency. It has the disadvantage, however, of limiting the flow of knowledge between personnel in the various disciplines.

Nursing home patients are served best in those facilities which discourage IABs. The satisfaction of their needs requires the concern and involvement of all staff members, regardless of the discipline with which they identify. The responsibilities of all employees overlap, and all are obligated to assist in attaining the goals set by every department. Thus, all staff members should expect, from time to time, to perform duties regularly executed by people assigned to disciplines different from their own.

Administrators sometimes fail to break down IABs, as when they avoid taking action to resolve personnel conflicts, disagreements, and other incidents demonstrating a lack of employee cooperation. For example, staff members who echo the phrase, "It's not my responsibility," when they are called upon to do something they think is not part of their job are reflecting an administrative tolerance of the IAB condition. IAB thinking is present when professionals fail to pick up paper or other objects from the floor because they view this as the task of houseworkers; when kitchen personnel fail to converse with patients because they fear criticism for acting out the role of nurses; when recreation activities personnel cannot get help to move patients to and from activity areas; when nurses' aides leave food droppings on wheelchairs for houseworkers to remove; and when office workers remove themselves completely from the lives of the patients and their families. Only when IAB attitudes are removed from the nursing home environment do the patients receive maximum care and service. They should be able to depend on the cooperative efforts of everyone to satisfy all their needs.

The Absence of Meaningful Sanitation Standards

Incontinence, the loss of control over the discharge of body waste, is a tough problem for nursing homes. It is the source of offensive odors which sometimes permeate the patient areas and create a most depressing environment. Most of the complaints registered against homes are related to this condition and, when it is detected by the general public, the image and reputation of these facilities are severely damaged.

There are times when it is particularly difficult to prevent unpleasant odors from coming into the nursing home environment. This is when there are more than the usual numbers of patients ill with bladder or bowel diseases, or during certain hours of the morning when the body functions of many people are active. Normally, however, odors from these conditions are temporary. It is when odors linger and are constant that the facility has sanitation problems. This is an indication that the facility is poorly managed and that the housekeeping procedures are inappropriate, infrequent, or sporadic. Odors come from bacteria, which collect on flat surfaces, mainly floors, bedding, windowsills, table tops, and similar places.

Nursing homes are not entirely to blame for these unsanitary conditions. They receive very little advice and direction from health agencies about proper techniques for controlling and eliminating them. Since there are no meaningful standard regulatory guidelines to assist the housekeeping personnel, masking agents (air fresheners), which serve only to cover up the odors caused by bacteria, are widely used. No specifications govern the kinds, or application, of sanitizing chemicals, and there are no health agency checks to ensure that what is used will kill even serious, infection-causing bacteria. In my 16 years as an administrator, no one ever questioned how the housekeeping procedures were carried out or what the bacteria killing power of the chemical agents used were. Under these circumstances, it is noteworthy that most homes have effective odor control programs even though they do not have the built-up technical expertise that more sophisticated kinds of health facilities have.

The Absence of Pertinent Education and Training for Nursing Home Personnel

Because nursing homes have not been recognized as a viable and skilled part of the health system, the training of health professionals has centered around the acute, technical aspects of care. This is so even though there are more patients in nursing homes than in acute general hospitals. Colleges, universities, and training schools have, therefore, geared most all of their health related career development programs to every sector of the health system except long term care. This goes far to account for the persistence of some inappropriate care concepts in nursing homes.

The most outstanding educational effort directed toward

nursing homes is focused on nursing home administrators, who are, by the way, the only health administrators to be licensed. They are required to receive from 20 to 40 hours of formal education and training each year to maintain their right to practice nursing home administration. Since the licensing program started in 1971, nursing home administrators have become the most trained administrators in the entire health system. Not surprisingly, the by-product of this effort has been a significant improvement in the quality of care delivered in homes throughout the country.

Educating administrators alone, however, is not enough to ensure quality care and services. They are generally removed from their facility's moment-to-moment and day-to-day activities, and do not always observe the care procedures used. If, as very often happens, they do not pass down to operational level personnel the philosophies, concepts, and subject matter they have studied, their training has been wasted. Some administrators attend training programs for the sole purpose of satisfying the training requirements and with no intention of transmitting what they have learned to the staffs of their facilities. Understandably, this is particularly likely to occur when the individual does not have the teaching experience or skill to act in the capacity of an instructor.

The most serious deficiency exists with respect to the pre-training and in-house training of nursing home operational level employees, i. e., nurses, nurses' aides, houseworkers, kitchenworkers, and so on. Ongoing educational courses are seldom offered by colleges, universities, or health agencies to train these people *specifically* for nursing home work. Most individuals who seek employment in these categories have had no related training. They may work in nursing homes for years without ever getting a formal introduction to the subjects of gerontology or long term care. Nurses' aides, the people who relate most directly to the patients, are usually hired off the streets without any understanding of the work they are expected to do. Many homes do not have personnel with teaching skills to thoroughly train people after they are hired. It is the failure of the nursing home and educational systems to develop meaningful training programs for operational level personnel that accounts for many of the sad experiences some patients have in homes. Until such time as educational institutions and health agencies promote special career development courses for every category of nursing home employee, the standard of service in some homes will not develop to the fullest.

Cost Controls that Limit Necessary Staffing

Ever since the early 1970s, a serious major effort has been carried out by exponents of health cost conservatism to redirect the health system and make it more fiscally responsible. This came about from a general awakening of society to the fact that the traditional ways of meeting our health needs were inefficient, wasteful of tax money, and failing to promote good health. Since this reform was directed toward the whole system, nursing homes fell prey to cost ceilings placed upon them by state rate-setting agencies which determine the daily service charges for publicly aided patients (the greater number of nursing home patients).

The experience nursing homes have had since the start of this cost-conscious period differs from that of acute-care hospitals. Those facilities have had a long history and have reached a point of maximum efficiency, and they deliver optimum service. They could readily adjust to strict fiscal controls and maintain their reputations for delivering quality care. The rapidly expanded and underdeveloped nursing home system, on the other hand, has not yet had enough time in which to refine its service procedures to the point where every home can be expected to deliver optimum service. Instead, these facilities are caused to operate under severe economic restraints while struggling to enhance their reputations.

Preceding sections of this book have explained what traditional nursing homes are like and have, through the experiences of an administrator-patient, empathized with patients and the experiences they have while living in those facilities. They have not only explored many of the conditions that cause patients to be deprived, but have also presented ideas and concepts useful in the effort to provide an environment which is conducive to a good quality of life for them. This particular chapter has focused on factors inherent in the system which complicate the task and hinder the efforts of homes to deliver the highest of quality care. A document of this kind would not be sincere or complete, however, if it did not offer solutions and methods to overcome the problems discussed. Part III presents some innovative educational and administrative concepts that are designed to assist homes in meeting their responsibility to deliver the best of patient care.

PART III

9

Inservice Training Concepts

Implementing effective administrative controls in a nursing home is more complex than it is in many other institutions or businesses. The very purpose for which the facility exists, and the nature of the work involved, present most difficult problems. Delivering care to older people is a sensitive responsibility requiring emotional concern on the part of every staff member, Some employees find it very rewarding; others find it depressing and hard to accept. Unusual stress situations, brought on by pressures associated with the work, can cause the morale of the personnel to change from moment to moment and from day to day. To deal with these conditions, the administration must be conscious of all of the dynamics taking place in the environment and employ measures which will foster common understandings about the patients' needs and the techniques that are used to reach the goals of the facility.

The inservice training concepts and techniques presented in this chapter will help to facilitate the delivery of optimum care by standardizing nursing home service modes. In addition, they will reduce the number of conflicts which develop among staff personnel, because the goals will be understood and there will be unity of purpose.

For these concepts to be effective and productive, they should be introduced to every staff member in a formal inservice training program and then, in order to keep the ideas alive, repeated or alluded to by department heads on a regular basis and whenever departmental meetings are held. All too frequently, the subject matter of inservice training sessions is never discussed again, and the time and effort involved with running the program is wasted. By frequent repetition, the concepts and modes will automatically become part of the systems and procedures used to care for the patients, and the terminology involved will become part of the language used in the home. The end result will be a staff that thoroughly understands its responsibilities and is interested in delivering superior care.

The material in this chapter is presented in simple terms and includes basic, essential management concepts so personnel will understand how a nursing home functions. It also includes care delivery concepts which will encourage the staff to recognize, respect, and service the patients' basic human needs. Most any responsible staff member has the capacity to interpret this material and deliver it to other personnel in a classroom setting. It is offered with the premise that educating nursing home staff members is vital if patients are to have a good quality of life.

I. Communication

An effective means of communicating between management and operational level personnel* is essential if the operation of the

---

* The term "operational level personnel" is used in this book instead of the term "lower level employees" because it is more respectful and also because it indicates the important responsibilities that these people have. It refers to those employees who function under the supervision of department heads.

nursing home is to be successful. This makes it possible to solidify the organization and meld it into one efficient unit. Without a good communication system, misconceptions develop among staff members. They develop feelings of insecurity, become preoccupied with rumors, and experience a lowering of morale.

A good communication network should provide for the transmittal of messages, sent periodically and consistently, from the administration to every member of the staff. This can be done through the issuance of bulletins, newsletters, or inhouse newspapers. The process should be supplemented by periodic meetings of all personnel, including the administrator. The subject matter of the communications should focus on all of the policies affecting the operation of the nursing home and on future plans for the facility. It should inform the staff of planning goals set by top management; convey information about special issues; and clarify and justify the personnel and operating policies put into effect by the administration.

No communication network can be successful if it does not provide for reverse transmission, interchange, and feedback. This means that anyone who receives a message can question it or seek clarification of its contents. The questioning, or interchange, may be initiated by anyone in the organization through his or her immediate supervisor. It may be in either written or verbal form. The use of a centrally placed box in which written questions and suggestions can be placed to be transmitted to the administrator is an effective means of soliciting ideas and feedback. The administrator has an obligation to respond to every signed inquiry and to consider unsigned notes carefully, since they might alert him to a problem that merits some action.

II. Understanding What a Good Quality of Life Means

As was stated on page 3 2, the term "quality of life," when applied to nursing home patients, refers to how well their environments satisfy their basic human needs. These include not only their physical-medical needs but also their social and psychological needs, particularly those analyzed in Chapter 3 of this book, i.e., possessions, freedom, privacy, independence, and all the others. For example, if the patients receive good medical care in addition to having their other basic needs satisfied, their quality of life may be considered good. If, however, the medical care is good but the patients are deprived of some of the other basic human needs, their quality of life is not what it should be.

All nursing home personnel should be conscious of what a good quality of life for their patients means. The manner in which they serve the patients will either enhance or defeat the purpose of using it as a goal. For example, if the patients are not given decision-making opportunities, or if they are denied freedom and independence when the potential exists for satisfying those needs, then their quality of life is lowered.

Providing a good quality of life for patients should serve as the foundation for implementing all the nursing home systems and procedures. It should be the underlying consideration during discussions, meetings, inservice training programs, and any time decisions are made which affect the operation of the nursing home. The question, "Do our policies and service delivery modes enable our patients to satisfy their basic human needs?" should always be on the mind of the administrator.

III. Understanding Nursing Home Management Functions

Management has the responsibility of directing the activities of a business or institution. Its functions are discussed here because it is important for every nursing home staff member to understand how management functions to govern the activities taking place in their facility and to gain some insight into the responsibilities of the administration. Most importantly, when staff members are familiar with these functions, they are better equipped to organize their work and carry out their duties in an efficient manner.

There are six nursing home management functions. They are presented here in an abbreviated form. Those who would like more information and discussion on management can find a good deal of literature on the subject in any public library. The six functions are:

1. *Planning Strategy.* Making plans for the future and setting goals so the home will maintain a high standard of patient care. The goals may be short-term or long-term. *Short-term goals* are those which are to be attained in a short period of time—the next day, the next week, the next month, and so on. *Long-term goals* are to be attained at some predetermined distant date. They are usually a year or more in the future.

2. *Organizing the Home.* Dividing the facility into different units, parts, or departments. The divisions are determined on the basis of the kinds of service given in the home. The traditional nursing home units include Administration, Nursing Service, Social Service, Kitchen, Housekeeping, Recreational Services, and so on. Each unit has a leader or department head.

3. *Staffing the Home.* Doing what is necessary to have enough people working in each unit so that the best of care and services will be given the patients.

4. *Procuring Resources.* Doing what is necessary to have enough materials and supplies in the home at all times.

5. *Supervising.* Instructing and advising others, most always subordinates, how best to discharge their responsibilities.

6. *Maintaining Control.* Establishing operating procedures which will foster a high level of personnel performance and patient care. The procedures are designed so that someone in the organization will be alerted when something goes wrong so that corrective action will be taken immediately. Control may be maintained by observing personnel and

through routine written monitoring reports (accounting statements, staffing reports, and so on) which are submitted to department heads or representatives of the administration for review.

These functions are almost always viewed as the responsibilities of administrators and not of operational level personnel. For nursing homes, however, this idea is false. There they are the responsibility of every single member of the nursing home staff. For example, nurses, nurses' aides, houseworkers, kitchenworkers, and others perform these functions when they plan and organize their work, keep their supervisors informed about staff conditions, check to be certain they have the proper amounts and kinds of materials and supplies, supervise or encourage colleagues to do their work well, and control their own work detail so that a high standard of performance is maintained. The six functions are guides which can help everyone plan and schedule their daily duties.

IV. Understanding the Meaning of Authority, Responsibility, and Influence

All nursing home personnel should thoroughly understand and be aware of the meanings of responsibility, authority, and influence. Such awareness will help to foster a spirit of cooperation among staff members, eliminate staff conflicts, and instill staff pride by giving employees an understanding of their positions within the organization and their roles in the patient care process.

Authority: This is the leadership power staff members have which enables them to place demands upon other employees. The number of people they can give orders to differs according to their position. For example, the administrator normally has the most power because he or she can enforce directives and give orders to anyone working in the home. Operational level personnel have less authority because fewer, if any, people report to them.

Authority is something that can be transferred to others. This is called *delegating authority*. It can only be transferred, however, by someone higher up in the organization than the person it is being delegated to. In other words, it is always relayed from higher positions in the home downward through the organization to the operational level staff members. *It cannot flow upward through the organization.* Understanding the dynamics of authority makes it clear that each person *has just one boss!* Any organization that does not define the order of authority for the staff is not well run. The following chart graphically shows how the line of authority should run in a nursing home.

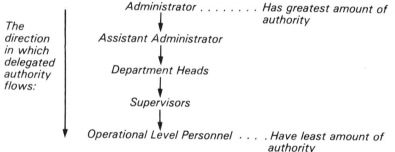

A Simplified Organizational Chart Showing the Line of Authority in a Nursing Home

Responsibility: This is the extent to which a staff member obligates himself or herself to carry out his or her assigned duties correctly and efficiently. It is also the extent to which a person can be relied upon by a superior to perform those duties well.

Differentiating Between Authority and Responsibility: Authority *can* be delegated to another person. Responsibility *cannot* be delegated because it is something a person assumes and takes upon himself or herself. Therefore, one person cannot make another person responsible. If the nursing home staff understands the meaning of these two terms, personnel conflicts will be avoided and utterances such as, "It's not my responsibility," will be discouraged.

Influence: Influence is a unique management concept especially appropriate for the operation of nursing homes. When used properly, it fosters and perpetuates quality nursing home care and services.

Influence means having a say about how the patients' care and services are delivered in the home. If patients are to enjoy a good quality of life in a nursing home, every staff member must be able to exercise influence by offering suggestions, expressing opinions, and making recommendations to improve the delivery of care and services. Operational level personnel, in particular, must be a part of this influence process. They often know the patients' intimate concerns better than those in higher positions and should make their knowledge known to those who have the authority to institute service procedures. This can be done during group discussions and meetings, during personal meetings with superiors, and at case discussion meetings. It should be an ongoing mode in the facility for the staff to show their interest in the well-being of the patients. Without the advice and counsel of operational level personnel, many basic human needs of patients will go unsatisfied. Influence, therefore, must travel both *up and down* throughout the entire nursing home if optimum patient care is to be provided. The following chart graphically shows how influence should flow in a home.

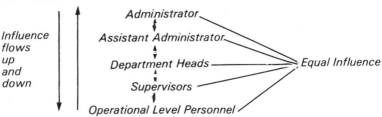

A Simplified Organizational Chart Showing how Influence Flows in a Nursing Home

V. Understanding how Basic Housekeeping and Sanitation Techniques Control Bacteria and Offensive Odors

Health facility sanitation, the science of which odor control is only a part, is very technical and complex. Books have been written on the subject and experts spend many years studying it. What is presented here is simplified and brief. The ideas and recommendations covered, however, will give nursing home personnel a basic knowledge of health facility sanitation and enable homes to eliminate unpleasant odors from their environment.* Most everyone working in long term care institutions—and particularly housekeeping personnel—should become familiar with the sanitation and cleaning data explained here.

When offensive odors are constantly present in a nursing home, it means that inappropriate cleaning techniques are being used. Sometimes it is an indication that the administration is delinquent by employing an insufficient number of housekeeping personnel.

The common sources of offensive odors in nursing homes are urine and the bacteria associated with patients' feces which may have been deposited in bedding, on the floor, on other surfaces, or temporarily stored in soiled linen-holding areas. Eliminating the resulting odors and potentially harmful disease-causing bacteria from the facility requires a methodical, frequent, and persistent cleaning effort.

Characteristics of Bacteria and Cleaning Agents

Some understanding of bacteria is basic for anyone having housekeeping responsibilities in nursing homes. They should know what they are, what they do, and what can be done to control them. If housekeeping personnel do not have this knowledge, it is likely that incorrect cleaning procedures will be used with the result that odors will stay in the environment.

---

* The books, *Hospital Sanitation—An Administrative Program* and *Food Service Sanitation* by Bertha Litsky, published by Modern Hospital Press, Chicago, Illinois, are recommended as necessary sources for a more in-depth study of this subject.

Bacteria are microorganisms (tiny living things) that can only be seen under powerful microscopes. They feed on dirt, multiply rapidly, can be transported from place to place by human beings or on moveable objects, and may even float through the air on dust particles. Some kinds of bacteria cause humans to become infected with serious diseases. It is the accumulation of these organisms in the nursing home environment that causes offensive odors.

Keeping the environment free of bacteria requires the use of many kinds of cleaning agents. Some may be detergents which are used to wash dirt away and have no bacteria killing or inhibiting properties. Others are formulated with special chemicals which will control bacteria. Each one, however, is manufactured to be used in specific places and for particular purposes. Care should be exercised when they are used. An agent which is recommended for use on floors, for example, may not be suitable for use on over-the-bed tables and other objects that are touched by the patients and staff. In all likelihood it would be an irritant to human skin.

It is extremely important that housekeeping personnel *do not* intermix one brand or type of chemical with another. It is conceivable that a toxic vapor or other harmful kind of chemical would result.

Cleaning agents should only be used in accordance with the directions shown on the container labels or use-instruction sheets. This data should tell where they are to be used, how they are to be used, and, importantly, the strains of organisms they will control. If this information about an agent is not available, then it is not worth running the risk of using it.

When purchasing a sanitizing agent, care should be exercised to determine if it is a bactericide, bacteriostat, or sporicide. *Bactericides,* as the word implies, will kill specific kinds of bacteria, whereas *bacteriostats* will only inhibit their growth. *Sporicides* are formulated to kill the most resistant kinds of bacteria—the spore-forming types that are encased in a protective film. Housekeepers who are unaware of the differences between these types of agents often believe that the cleaning agents they use will kill disease-causing organisms when, in fact, they will not. This underscores the importance of knowing what the chemicals are and what they will do so the cleaning procedures can be scientific, consistent, and thorough.

Many kinds of cleaning agents have dual or even multiple qualities. An agent may be a detergent-disinfectant, a detergent-bacteriostat-bactericide, or other combination of chemicals. The labels on the containers and/or the use-instruction sheets should always specify what the agents are and the kinds of bacteria they will control.

Recommended Procedures for Controlling Bacteria and Odors

The floors of the nursing home, particularly in those areas used by incontinent patients, are prime collecting points for bacteria and related offensive odors. The facility will not be free of this condition unless a persistent effort is made to keep the floors clean and sanitized. If this is not done, bacteria will be picked up on peoples' shoes and tracked throughout the home. They may also be transferred to the hands of people who retrieve objects that have been dropped on the floor. The following procedures are recommended to control bacteria and odors.

Floors

1. Floors should be mopped *daily.*
2. A cleaning agent, or agents, having detergent and bacteria killing power should be used.
3. Accidental spillage or dropping of human waste should be picked up and sanitized immediately upon notice of this condition. Every staff member should take whatever action is necessary to ensure that the waste is removed promptly.

4. Mop heads used on floors should be washed separately in a washing machine and dried separately in a clothes dryer after each use. A clean mop head should be used for every fresh pail of cleaning fluid. A contaminated mop head will contaminate newly replenished cleaning fluids.

5. There should be frequent replenishing of the cleaning agent. The square footage area being cleaned per bucket, as recommended by the manufacturer, should be strictly followed.

6. The floors of holding areas where laundry baskets containing soiled linen are stored should receive special attention. This room is a significant source of odors.

7. During late hours when the regular housekeeping staff is not working, special arrangements should be made so that cleaning chemicals and equipment are available for use. There should always be personnel designated to clean unusual contaminating conditions.

Other Flat Surfaces

1. All flat surfaces in the facility should be cleaned daily. These areas include table tops, over-the-bed tables, chairs, bureaus, windowsills, cabinets, counter tops, and other surfaces.

2. When over-the-bed tables are used by patients for feedings, they should be wiped before and after every meal. A nonirritating sanitizing agent should be used.

3. Nonirritating-type sanitizing chemicals should be used for all flat surfaces which might be touched by the patients or staff members. Bacteriostat agents may be used.

4. Flat surfaces in soiled linen holding areas should not be overlooked.

5. These procedures apply to every room in the facility, i. e., lounges, bedrooms, nursing stations, activities rooms, kitchen, corridors, libraries, offices, etc.

Interior Walls and Windows

1. Bedroom walls, corridor walls, and other walls which may be touched by the patients and staff should be wiped with a sanitizing agent at least every two weeks.
2. A detergent and disinfectant or a combination detergent-disinfectant should be used.
3. Inside window glass should be cleaned at least every week.
4. An appropriate window cleaner with sanitizing qualities should be used on glass.
5. The facility should have a scheduled program for a thorough cleaning effort throughout the environment four times a year.

Toilet Areas

1. Toilet areas should receive a thorough cleaning on the 7 A.M. to 3 P.M. and 3 P.M. to 11 P.M. shifts.
2. There should be monitoring of the toilet areas by a designated staff member on the 11 P.M. to 7 A.M. shift and arrangements should be made to remove accidental contamination during these hours.
3. Nonirritating disinfectant type chemical agents should be used.
4. Air fresheners should not be relied upon to remove odors in toilet areas.

Soiled Linen and Patients' Clothes

1. The bedsheets, blankets, mattresses, and clothing of incontinent patients should be monitored for soilage at one-hour intervals or less, depending upon the physical condition of the patients.
2. Patients should be encouraged to notify a member of the staff whenever they need bladder or bowel attention. These requests for service should be responded to promptly.

3. When soiled linen or clothing is detected, it should be replaced immediately. Appropriate skin care, utilizing reputable powders or lotions, should be applied to the patients promptly.
4. Soiled linen should not be allowed to touch the floor. This is to prevent further accumulation of bacteria on the floor.
5. Soiled linen and clothing should be placed immediately in laundry hampers having disposable plastic bag liners.
6. The liners should then be tied at the top to seal in offensive odors.
7. The hamper should then be taken to the holding area or laundry department to await washing.

NOTES: Caring for incontinent patients and handling their soiled garments and bedding are the most difficult of all problems associated with nursing homes. It takes a persistent effort on the part of the staff to overcome the odor difficulties associated with incontinence. No other problems, however, deserve more attention than these do. A methodical program to service patients with this disability will not only safeguard them but it will also safeguard the staff, families, and other visitors. It will also preserve the reputation of the facility.

Air fresheners *should not* be considered a means of controlling odors. They only mask the condition and do not remove bacteria from the environment. Their use should be restricted to what might be considered emergency situations.

VI. Looking at Patients and Their Needs from a Different Perspective

If the question, "What are nursing homes supposed to do for patients?" was asked of a group of nursing home administrators, the responses would be quite varied. Hopefully, one of them would have read this book and would respond, "To give them a good quality of life." Even this response is unclear, however, because it does not fully explain what a good quality of life is or indicate how to accomplish that objective.

The fact of the matter is that nursing homes are supposed to care for elderly people just as the heads of a household care for their family members—the responsibilities are the same, i.e., to provide support and service that are conducive to a long, healthy, and peaceful life. The ingredients for such a life are:

- Good nutrition
- Exercise
- Freedom from anxiety and stress
- Freedom from accidents
- Freedom from disease and physical disabilities

These are listed below along with suggested measures for attaining them in nursing homes.

Nutrition

1. A certified dietitian should monitor the meals of every patient.
2. The dietitian should counsel patients who overeat as well as those who undereat.
3. The home should serve balanced meals:
   - Meat and fish for protein
   - Fruits for vitamins and minerals (citrus fruits for vitamin C)
   - Vegetables for vitamins, minerals, and bulk
   - Dairy products for calcium
   - Wheat and grains for carbohydrates and fiber
4. Serving excessive amounts of refined carbohydrates should be avoided.
5. Serving excessive amounts of red meats should be avoided.
6. Chicken and fish should be served as often as, or even more often than, red meats.
7. Milk and fruit juices should be available at every meal.
8. Consumption of excessive amounts of coffee and tea should be discouraged.

9. There should be a variety of special nutritious diets available for those patients who cannot eat regular meals.
10. The patients should be educated about good eating habits and foods essential to their good health.
11. The home should endeavor to educate patients' families about nutrition.

NOTE: Number 1 above is vital. A good nutrition program depends upon the skill of a qualified dietitian.

Exercise
1. The patients' attending physicians should issue exercise authorizations.
2. Patients should exercise within their physical limits *daily*. Those who can walk should be encouraged to do so every day. Wheelchair and bed patients should do range of motion exercises daily.

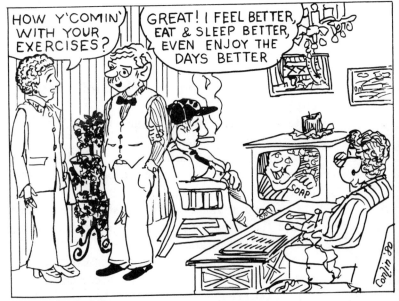

EXERCISES....

3. The home should have an outside exercise area, complete with walkways and appropriate exercise devices.
4. A simplified record system should be devised so that the consistency of each patient's exercising regimen can be monitored.
5. The exercise program should be considered a recreational activity and should be part of the recreational activities program.

Freedom from Anxiety and Stress

1. An empathetic attitude on the part of the staff toward patients will remove some of the patients' anxieties.
2. Patients should be encouraged to express their concerns freely to someone on the staff whom they trust.
3. The staff and, in particular, the social worker, should respond to patients' concerns quickly.
4. There should be ongoing efforts to encourage family visits.
5. Families should be made aware of the dynamics of anxiety and stress and should be encouraged to respond to the patients' concerns.
6. Visits from clergymen should be encouraged.
7. Patients should be given prompt assistance when they exhibit a desire to communicate with people outside of the home.
8. The facility should have a good recreational activities program, not only for arts and crafts, but also for activities that encourage patient and staff group interaction.

Fredom from Accidents

1. The home should have a good safety program.
2. The patients should be protected from walking on slippery floors.
3. There should be adequate lighting in patient-use areas at all times.

4. Equipment and other objects should not be left in corridors and other areas where patients walk.
5. Smoking by patients should be in controlled areas only.

Freedom, as Much as Possible, from Disease and Physical Disabilities

1. The home should have enough nurses to schedule at least four hours of nursing time per day per patient.
2. Physician consultation and service should be readily available for each patient.
3. The home should have adequate medical equipment.
4. The home should have the services of a reliable and prompt pharmacy.
5. Medications should be under the strict control of a registered nurse.
6. Procedures should be employed to avoid prescribing and distributing unnecessary medications.
7. There should be ongoing inservice training programs for the nursing staff.
8. Maintenance therapy disciplines such as physiotherapy, speech therapy, occupational therapy, and recreational activity therapy should be available to patients as needed.
9. Emergency hospital service should be readily available.
10. The home should have an efficient and reliable source for laboratory testings.
11. The facility should have a good housekeeping and infection control program.
12. The cleaning chemicals used in the facility should be appropriate for the task involved and be under strict control.

VII. Inservice Training Concepts to Standardize Operational Goals and Objectives

This section presents inservice educational concepts that are essential for training nursing home personnel in every category. The concepts are comprehensive in scope and fundamental to the delivery of quality nursing home care and services. Study and discussion of this material will stimulate the staff's interest in and concern for older patients. As the staff gains greater empathetic appreciation for the elderly people they serve, they will become more highly motivated to help them overcome their deprivations. Service delivery modes will become standardized, the staff will become unified, and the care discipline most appropriate for nursing homes will be clarified.

The Dynamics of Patients' Sensory Deprivations

It is through the senses of *seeing, hearing, smelling, tasting, and touching* that we perceive our environments. When these elements are combined with our memories, experiences, emotions, and thoughts, they determine how we relate and react to our environment. If, for example, the acuity of one or more of our senses is reduced or lost, our perceptions of our surroundings are distorted. This can cause us to be deprived of opportunities for enjoying the normal activities of daily living. A total loss, particularly the loss of sight or hearing, may cause extreme feelings of anxiety and emotional stress which may eventually manifest itself in a variety of physical illnesses.

All service delivery personnel, particularly nurses and nurses' aides, should thoroughly understand and always be aware of the dynamics of sensory loss. It is a condition which not only contributes toward people's physical decline but also affects their psychological well-being. For instance, it can affect staff/patient, patient/patient, and patient/family relationships. Most significantly, it frequently causes patients to become confused, withdrawn, depressed, and disoriented. For the purpose of helping nursing home personnel recognize the results of patients' sensory losses, the common characteristics associated with them are listed below.

Common Characteristics of Vision Loss

1.   Patients may have difficulty focusing eyes.

2.   Adjustment to light may decline.
3.   Adaptation to darkness may be slowed down (night blindness).
4.   Patients may find it strange when reaching for things, i.e., they may not be able to quite reach what they are trying to pick up.
5.   Sensitivity to color contrasts may be reduced.
6.   Peripheral vision (seeing things from the right or left of direct sight) may be impaired.

Common Characteristics of Hearing Loss

1.   Men show a greater incidence of hearing loss than women do.
2.   With hearing loss, men hear low frequencies best; women hear high frequencies best.
3.   Patients may not be able to identify certain noises.
4.   Patients may misinterpret noises.
5.   Patients may be sensitive to vibrations within the environment.

Common Characteristics of Taste Loss

1.   Taste buds lose sensitivity.
2.   Patients may not be able to differentiate between foods which have similar tastes.
3.   Patients may want highly seasoned foods and sweets because they can taste them.
4.   Some patients may complain that the food is too bland.

Common Characteristics of Sense of Smell Loss

1.   Patients are unable to detect most odors in the environment; they may not be conscious of their own odors.
2.   Since part of the pleasure of eating comes from smelling food, some patients have a loss of appetite.

Common Characteristics of Sensory Change of Touch

1. Patients' finger sensitivity may decline and some patients may drop things.
2. Some patients may be more sensitive to cold and may need to wear extra clothing.
3. Some patients may be more sensitive to heat.

Our senses are interrelated and interdependent. Several of them are involved in every contact we have with our environment. For example, to fully appreciate a rose, one must be able to see it, smell it, and touch it. To fully enjoy food, one must see it, smell it, and taste it. Therefore, when the acuity of one of the senses is reduced, the opportunity for the full enjoyment of some experiences is reduced. Enjoyment can be enhanced, however, by increased acuity of the less affected senses. Blind people, for instance, rely more than ever on their hearing.

Nursing home personnel who understand the interrelatedness of the senses can help patients compensate for their sensory losses. The following material lists some things the staff can do.

How the Staff Can Help Patients Compensate for Loss of Visual Acuity

1. If alert patients are unable to read any longer, speak to them about the events happening in world affairs, sports, and so on.
2. Speak clearly at a volume patients can comfortably hear.
3. Encourage patients to touch objects and materials and to figure out what they are.
4. Give partially-sighted patients reading material that has large print.
5. Tell patients what is on their food tray. Do not take it for granted that they can see what they are eating.

6. Approach patients directly from the front. They may not be able to see things from the side of their vision.
7. Encourage patients to listen to the radio. Help them locate programs that interest them. Make a list of these programs and the times and stations they are on and remind patients to tune in to them.
8. Tell patients the time as often as necessary.
9. Help patients write letters and use a phone.
10. Help patients maintain their radios.
11. Talk about the kinds and colors of clothing they and the other patients are wearing.
12. Stimulate conversations among the patients.
13. Tell patients what the weather is like each day.
14. Show love by laying hands on the patients.

How the Staff Can Help Patients Compensate for Loss of Hearing Acuity

1. Speak slowly and clearly at a volume the patients can comfortably hear.
2. Face the patients directly when talking to them so they will have the opportunity to lip read.
3. Encourage patients to touch, taste, smell, and see objects existing in the environment.
4. Explain unusual or loud noises.
5. Explain unusual vibrations in the environment.
6. Do not ignore patients when they do not speak first.
7. Find interesting reading material for alert patients.
8. Keep pad and pencil handy so you can write your communication if necessary.
9. Encourage patients to watch TV programs that interest them.
10. Show love by laying hands on the patients.

How the Staff Can Help Patients Compensate for Loss of Taste Acuity

1. Tell patients what they are eating and how it was prepared.
2. Identify the meats, vegetables, fruits, and fish when they are being served.
3. Offer the patients condiments if that is appropriate.
4. Allow them to sample different treats if appropriate.

How the Staff Can Help Patients Compensate for Loss of Sense of Smell

1. Encourage patients to smell certain identifiable foods as they eat.
2. Encourage patients to smell flowers, perfumes, herbs, and spices.
3. Talk to patients about things that have identifiable scents.

How the Staff Can Help Patients Compensate for Changes in Sense of Touch

1. Encourage patients to feel objects and fabrics.
2. Respond to patients' concerns over heat and cold.
3. Guard patients against exposure to excessively hot or cold water during their baths or showers.
4. Be sympathetic when patients drop things.

It is recommended that discussions be encouraged during inservice training programs and at meetings to explore the dynamics associated with sensory loss. Ideas about possible measures to compensate for these losses should be solicited from all staff members, particularly nurses' aides because they have the most contact with the patients. Awareness of how sensory losses affect patients should be part of the daily service delivery modes and part of every inservice training program. An effort of this kind will sponsor empathetic feelings on the part of the staff toward the patients.

An Effective Awareness Program

The awareness program presented here is an extension of the methods that were recommended to compensate for sensory deprivations. It considers an additional dimension that contributes directly to patients' loss of contact with reality and to their unreal perceptions of their environments. This dimension is their *dissociation* from familiar experiences, clues, links, or reminders necessary for self-awareness. Stated simply, this means that when older people find themselves living in an unnatural nursing home environment, removed from things they knew in the past, they may become more forgetful. In extreme cases they may become mentally confused and disoriented.

Forgetfulness is not always something indigenous to old age. Everyone forgets details and things that have happened to them in the past. Middle-aged people, for example, find it impossible to recall many of the meaningful events and happy times of their early childhood because they have been disengaged from those experiences for so many years. If people had continual daily reminders of their early youth through their middle years, they would be able to recall and relive those experiences.

Dissociation, which is often compounded by physiological changes in the brain and by depression, induces pronounced forgetfulness on the part of nursing home patients. They can lose interest in and forget even the most elementary things. They may become unaware of the time, the date, the reality of the environment in which they live, and their past histories, including their relationship with members of their own families. This phenomenon is often explained by the term "senility," or attributed to organic brain damage. Frequently, however, it can be alleviated by effective recall techniques.

The concepts used in a nursing home awareness program are modifications of the popular reality orientation and remotivation techniques. It differs from them because it does not sponsor the use of specially designed props or advocate formal staff/patient group sessions. Because those kinds of efforts place excessive time demands upon the staff, they often fall by the wayside and are eventually abandoned.

The awareness program is introduced to the nursing home staff during inservice training sessions. When enforced, it becomes part of the everyday, 24-hour mode of servicing the patients. It is carried out through natural, regular conversations which take place between staff members and patients while routine care is being delivered. It is a method whereby nurses and others recognize the patients' sensory losses and their dissociation from reality, and seize every opportunity to remind them of clues which will link them with the real environment and their past experiences. In other words, the patients' recall powers are stimulated. The only extra effort involves the use of a "patient profile sheet," prepared by social service personnel, which contains nonconfidential histories of the patients. The steps needed for an awareness program follow.

How to Implement an Effective Awareness Program

1. Include the awareness program subject in inservice training sessions and require all newly employed staff members to be introduced to its methods soon after they begin working. Review the topic three or four times a year so the technique will be ongoing. Enforce the idea that this system is part of the nursing home care discipline.
2. When conducting inservice programs covering this subject, enlarge upon the material in the first three paragraphs in this section (pages 162 and 163). The entire staff

Patient Profile Sheet

Name_____Date of birth_____Age___
Male____Female____Nationality_____Date of admittance___
Married_____Single_____Widowed_____
Birthplace_____Languages spoken_____
First name of spouse or former spouse (if any)_____
Former occupation of patient_____

Names of sons and daughters	Occupations and special accomplishments of sons and daughters
_____	_____
_____	_____
_____	_____
_____	_____

Names of parents, brothers, sisters	Occupations and special accomplishments of parents, brothers, and sisters
_____	_____
_____	_____
_____	_____
_____	_____
_____	_____
_____	_____

Special accomplishments of patient_____

Clubs or organizations belonged to_____

Likes_____Dislikes _____
Hobbies_____Special interests_____
Special experiences enjoyed in past_____
Places lived in_____
Places traveled to_____
Other meaningful facts or special history_____
_____
_____

should understand how dissociation contributes toward the patients' forgetfulness and disorientation.

3.   Develop a *patient profile sheet* for each patient. This form lists basic nonconfidential facts about each patient—his or her past endeavors, activities, occupations, special experiences, accomplishments, likes and dislikes, family history, and other significant data. When filling out the form, multiple copies should be made. The original should be placed on one clipboard and the duplicates on others. The clipboards should be hung in strategic locations such as the nurses' station and the kitchen. Since there will be as many profile sheets on each clipboard as there are patients on the unit, the sheets should be placed in alphabetical order, according to the patients' last names.

Every staff member should be required to read the profile sheets of new patients and to review those of other patients at regular intervals so they will become familiar with the backgrounds of every patient. They will then have a realistic knowledge of the patients and be better equipped to discuss topics of interest with them. This procedure will not only help the patients relate to their pasts, but will also give them much-needed recognition.

4.   The profile sheets should be prepared by the social service department after consultation with the patients and their families. This should be done for every patient at the time of admittance. Care should be exercised to be certain that information the families and the patients consider confidential will not be included on these forms.

5.   The staff should be informed that they are expected to use the following methods in the normal course of giving care to the patients:

   a.   Remind patients each day of the date, time, name of the facility, and their own name. This should be done in a normal and inconspicuous manner.

   b.   Seize every opportunity to talk to patients about subjects that are related to their past histories.

    c.   Seize every opportunity to talk to patients about things in the environment and about the weather outside.

    d.   Seize every opportunity to talk to patients about special holidays and birthdays.

    e.   Address patients by their accustomed names. Unless they ask to be called by a specific name, use the name they were known by before they came into the facility. Do not use newly applied nick names.

    f.   Talk to patients about nature and the seasons of the year.

    g.   Stimulate conversations among patients.

    h.   Use the techniques described on pages 159-161 for those who have sensory deprivations.

    i.   Run awareness program for families so they will learn about the awareness techniques, or invite them to the regular inservice training sessions. Educating families about sensory deprivation and awareness techniques will enhance the program. It will also make the families' visits more pleasurable for both family and patient.

6.   The following standard items will serve as aids to a good awareness program.

    a.   Large clock in each patient room.

    b.   Large calendar in each patient room.

    c.   Radios and TVs in patient rooms when practical.

    d.   Use of telephones when desired by the patients.

7.   The staff should be continually reminded to read and reread the profile sheets.

An awareness program has no leaders and involves no extra staff time since it takes place when staff personnel come in contact with patients. The techniques involved are strictly conversational and are designed to encourage the staff to recognize the patients as human beings and to stimulate the patients' recall powers. It is a method of reducing the patients' anxieties and making their lives more interesting and meaningful. Some of the times when the staff should use awareness techniques are:

> When patients awaken in the morning.
> When bathing or washing patients.
> When assisting patients onto chairs.
> When dressing patients.
> When grooming patients.
> When serving patients their meals.
> When making beds.
> When cleaning patients' rooms.
> When giving patients treatments.
> When giving patients their medications.
> When passing nourishments.
> When patients attend activity programs.
> When patients exercise.
> When sorting patients' clothes.
> When patients receive gifts from their families.
> When transporting patients on elevators.
> When assisting patients into bed.
> When answering night calls.
> When making special visits to patients for the specific purpose of talking to them.

VIII. The Nursing Home Philosophy

Every nursing home should have a well-thought-out and declared operational philosophy—a statement defining the purposes of the facility and its objectives. It is something that everyone working in the home should be aware of because it tells what the results of their efforts are expected to be. Two examples of nursing home philosophies are:

> The purposes of this nursing home are to deliver excellent medical care and to provide an environment which will enable patients to live peaceful, meaningful lives.

The purposes of this facility are to satisfy the physical, social, psychological, and environmental needs of patients and to serve their families.

A philosophy is not something to be printed in personnel manuals and then forgotten. It should be attractively printed and mounted and should be displayed in the lobby of the facility and in every servicing department. Thus, the staff will be constantly reminded of why the home is operated and what its objectives are. Posting the philosophy is also a means of telling families and visitors what the care standards of the home are.

Formulating Inservice Training Fundamentals

Having a well-constructed facility and good systems and procedures will not, by themselves, guarantee that the objectives of a nursing home will be attained. The work, attitudes, and actions of the staff will determine that. For instance, even though a patient's room is large enough for a reasonable number of possessions, the space is useless if personnel discourage belongings from coming into the institution. Likewise, talk about independence and freedom is meaningless if staff members thwart the patients by ignoring those needs.

Educational programs conducted in the nursing home should be designed to motivate the staff to satisfy the needs of patients to the maximum degree, and to prevent or compensate for patients' deprivations. Whether the training offered is about medical care, housekeeping, food service, or other topics, the needs that are important to the patients must be the primary concern. Understanding the dynamics of sensory deprivation, having an effective awareness program, and establishing a nursing home philosophy are fundamental elements in delivering good nursing home care.

The following two principles pull together all the concepts and considerations presented in this book. Understanding them should give staff members a greater awareness of, and appreciation for, the nursing home care discipline. Understanding the principles will also help to motivate staff members to meet their responsibilities and do whatever they can to help the patients satisfy their needs.

1.   Principle of Basic Human Needs Deprivation:
     Basic Human Needs Deprivation + Sensory Loss = Anxiety and Stress = Withdrawal = Disinterest, Confusion, Disorientation, Forgetfulness, Physical Decline

     OR: BHND + SL = AS = W = PPL (physical and psychological loss)

     Explanation: When patients' deprivations are compounded by their sensory losses, it causes them to experience anxiety and stress. This induces them to withdraw from the environment and undergo physical and psychological decline.

2.   Principle of Gerontological Environmental Dynamics:
     Empathy + Philosophy + Gerontological Environmental Dynamics + Management Functions = Patient Well-Being and a Good Quality of Life

     OR: E + P + GED + MF = WBQ

     Explanation: When the empathetic feelings of the staff (the foundation of good care) are motivated by the philosophy of the nursing home, and when the staff understands gerontological concepts and environmental factors, and when the management functions are designed to recognize the total needs of the patients, the patients' well-being and quality of life will be enhanced.

     Once these formulas are understood, they will clarify the discipline of nursing home care. They should be studied during inservice training and posted in strategic locations in the facility such as nursing stations. Supervisors should be required to discuss them from time to time. Periodic inquiries or formal testing will provide an indication of the staff's understanding of them.

10

Locating a Home and Admittance to a Home

What Constitutes A Good Home?
The customary method for families of potential nursing home patients to learn if a particular home delivers quality care is to observe the environment of the facility. They try to determine if the facility is free of offensive odors, if it serves good meals, if it conveys a pleasant atmosphere, and if it is fully licensed by state agencies. The premise is that, if a home looks good and has the necessary operating certificates, it follows that the patient care will be good. This is not necessarily so, however, because these indicators alone do not determine how patients are treated by the staff throughout the days and nights. It is the amount of compassionate attention the patients receive, and whether or not they are able to satisfy their basic human needs, that determine the quality of the services.

The following 12 care factors are more positive indicators of a good nursing home and will be helpful in finding a suitable facility for a loved one. They require that inquiries be made of staff members, patients, and the families of patients using the facility under consideration.

1. *Does the facility always have an offensive odor?*
   If the facility always has urine and feces' odors, that is a definite indication that the housekeeping is poor. Under such conditions, there is a strong possibility that infectious diseases could be present in the environment, creating a hazard to patients, staff, families, and visitors.

2. *Does the facility have a large enough nursing staff?*
   A good home will have a minimum staff ratio of at least 3.6 hours of nursing time (excluding supervisors) per patient per 24-hour day. This is determined by adding all the nursing hours of all the nursing personnel—RNs, LPNs, and nurses' aides—assigned over a 24-hour period and then dividing the total by the number of patients they serve. (Example: 360 nursing hours ÷ 100 patients = 3.6 hours). An adequate staff would be indicated by the following sample staffing patterns for each working shift.
   7 AM to 3 PM shift—average of one nurse to five patients
   3 PM to 11 PM shift—average of one nurse to seven patients
   11 PM to 7AM shift—average of one nurse to ten patients

3. *Is there a rapid turnover of the nursing staff?*
   Good homes have a relatively stable staff. This is an indication that the supervision is good and that the employees are satisfied with the working conditions.

4. *Do the patients get adequate nurse attention?*
   If a facility has a large enough nursing staff and the patients have to wait unreasonable amounts of time to have their needs attended to, it is an indication of poor supervision.

5. *Do the patients receive compassionate nursing care?*
   This can be determined by observing the attitudes of staff members and by asking patients and/or their families.

6. *Does the facility conduct regular inservice training programs for the staff and new employees?*
This is a *key indicator* of quality care. It means that the facility has set goals, recognizes the training needs of nursing home personnel, and is trying to deliver good care and services.

7. *Does the facility have adequate recreational personnel?*
A good facility will employ one full-time recreational person for approximately every 33 patients.

8. *Does the administrator remain aloof from the affairs of the home?*
A good home will have an administrator who will personally monitor all the activities of the facility. He or she will visit the patients regularly and converse with families to learn if they are satisfied with the care their relatives are receiving. The administrator will use his or her authority to correct deficiencies observed in the care systems.

9. *Are the meals appropriate and adequate?*
The home should serve balanced meals daily. The patients should receive fresh vegetables, fruits, chicken, and fish. The meals should be under the control of a competent and certified dietitian. The patients should receive adequate quantities of food. Heavy reliance on precooked and canned foods is not indicative of a well-run kitchen.

10. *Does the home have a good image in the community?*
Good homes have good reputations.

11. *Does the home have open visiting hours?*
Good homes appreciate visits from family members throughout the day and evening. Families that visit often and display interest in their elderly relatives can often influence the quality of care they receive.

12. *Do the patients go outside?*
In good homes, patients will be seen outside during pleasant weather. Staff members should be seen along with them.

The Patient Admittance Procedure

Admitting a relative to a nursing home is a most painful experience for both patients and their families. It is a climactic event which will force dramatic changes of lifestyles upon them. The patients sacrifice most all of their worldly possessions and pleasures, and the family members face the reality, accompanied by guilt feelings, that they can no longer provide care and comfort for their loved ones. Carrying out the admittance procedure in a sensitive manner is a nursing home responsibility.

Most people give little thought to the possibility that their mother or father will some day live in a nursing home. Usually, that idea is buried in their subconscious and covered over with the hope that some miracle will prevent it from happening. Most often, when it does become a reality, nothing has been planned to prepare for the transition. Little preparation may have been made to formulate property settlements, to arrange for payment of new financial obligations, or to the technicality of determining which family member will be responsible for handling all the connected personal and management affairs. Probably no thought has gone into the problem of just how the admittance will be handled.

Admittance to a nursing home is a contingency facing every American family, and should be thought about well in advance of the happening. Property transfers and other special financial matters should be resolved in a legal way while mother or father is well. It is best when this is done several years before the admittance takes place. If these arrangements are not made beforehand, the procedures for resolving them will become very complicated. Unnecessary legal expense will become part of the problem. Should the mental faculties of the admitted person be impaired, and he or she has property and financial holdings, the difficulties of managing these affairs can become awesome.

Once it becomes certain that mother or father must be admitted to a home, the procedure should be handled with great discretion. The rule, "Honesty is the best policy," applies. The person to be admitted should be told candidly that he or she is going to take up residency in a home. This, of course, precludes that this individual cannot make the decision alone. Statements such as, "You're going in for just a little while—we'll take you home as soon as we can," should be avoided. Older people are wise and know when their sons and daughters are not telling the truth. The following admittance statement was made to an older lady by her daughter, and it represents a good way of telling a loved one that he or she is to be admitted to a nursing home. Note that the last part of the statement offers a little hope.

> "Mother, you require so much care and attention now that we cannot take care of you at home any more. You're going to take up residency in the Hillview Nursing Home. You must understand, Mother, that it is unlikely that we will be able to bring you home, but if God makes you well enough, you know we will come for you. We will see you a lot, and we'll pray for you, because we want you with us."

When a patient enters a home for the first time, accompanied by family members, the administrator should see that everything possible is done to lighten their burdens. They are all suffering a great deal of emotional stress. The family should be encouraged to stay with the patient as long as possible. If possible, they should have the upcoming meal with the patient and remain by his or her side well into the evening. The whole staff of the facility should be aware that the newly admitted person is experiencing the "first night phenomenon."

Because the first few days are particularly stressful for newly admitted patients, a nurse or nurses' aide should be assigned (one on one) to stay with them as much as possible and give them priority attention for the first 48 hours. This will remove some of their anxieties and give them confidence in their new home.

It will also demonstrate to the families that the staff really cares and is concerned for the patients as human beings.

What Families Can Do for Patients

Nursing homes cannot, alone, satisfy all the needs of all the patients all the time. For them to receive the best of service and have their needs satisfied requires the involvement and cooperation of families. Sometimes families do not realize what they can do and wonder if it is permissible for them to help. They might even feel reluctant to interfere with the care process. The fact of the matter is that every bit of assistance they give benefits the patient greatly. It should be understood, however, by all members of the staff that when family members help patients, it does not remove the involved chore responsibility from the staff. The following list suggests some ways that families can help to care for their relatives when they visit the facility.

1. Take wearing apparel home to wash or have cleaned
2. Shine patient's shoes
3. Comb patient's hair
4. Clean patient's fingernails
5. Clean table tops and drawers
6. Clean dentures
7. Clean eyeglasses
8. Feed patient
9. Wash patient's hands
10. Walk with patient
11. Take patient outside
12. Assist during recreational programs
13. Take patient home for a day or weekend (*Note*: It is appropriate to use public assistance money—monthly subsistence allowance—for ambulance or van transportation)
14. Help with patient's exercises

15. Help with the application of cosmetics
16. Paint patient's fingernails
17. Visit other patients who have few visitors
18. Shave patient
19. Take patient out to a restaurant for a meal
20. Take patient to movies, concerts, or church (if practical)
21. Take patient home for a day
22. Take patient for a ride in an automobile

Suggested Gifts Families Might Bring Patients

1. Clothes, sweaters, slippers, and so on
2. Special sweets (if appropriate)
3. Clock with large numerals
4. Calendar with large print
5. Fruits (if appropriate)
6. Costume jewelry
7. Watch
8. Books
9. Magazine subscriptions
10. Newspaper subscription
11. Transistor radio
12. Cosmetics
13. Painting, knitting, or hobby kits
14. Puzzles
15. Toiletry items
16. Brush and combs
17. Perfume
18. Razor and shaving cream
19. Calculator
20. Belt
21. Shawl
22. Photographs and snapshots
23. Favorite foods (if appropriate)

11

Conclusions and Recommendations

The health system as it has evolved to serve elderly disabled people is in need of simplification. It consists of an uncoordinated conglomeration of facilities and services developed for individuals who are thought to have varying degrees of medical and social needs. All of them, including some not heretofore mentioned, such as retirement homes, congregate living facilities, and recently titled facilities called homes for frail elderly, provide some basic medical services, although their environments, operating procedures, and scope of services differ. Some even have nursing home units attached to them to deliver concentrated nursing and medical care. They all attempt, through differing viewpoints and approaches, to achieve the common objective of satisfying the needs of older people.

Good or bad, however, having so many varied health service entities tends, magnet-like, to pull older people out of society and segregate them. This is counter to the belief prevailing among many gerontologists that the health system should be structured to maintain people in their residences until concentrated nursing and medical care in an institution is necessary. It also induces a random movement of older people to and from society and among the many different kinds of facilities. The following illustration conceptualizes the current health system for older people in graphic form.

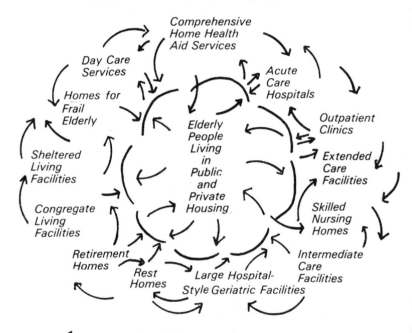

= Random movement of older people to and from society and among facilities and services

The Current Health System for Older People

Because nursing homes will continue to be relied upon to care for many disabled people, they are a key factor in developing a simplified comprehensive health care system for the elderly. This is true because the emerging trend to employ community-based home health aid services will never, for logistical and financial reasons, succeed in maintaining all older people in their residences. Before an effort to simplify the care system can succeed, however, nursing homes must embark on programs to improve their environments so they can more effectively satisfy the needs of their patients. Not to do so will perpetuate the current failures of these facilities and nullify their opportunity to become more viable. Most particularly, they must be changed to function under a single, uniform, and standardized set of government sponsored regulations which will remove the inequities and economic waste presently built into the long term care system. The following illustration visualizes the important role homes should play in a more simplified health care system for the future.

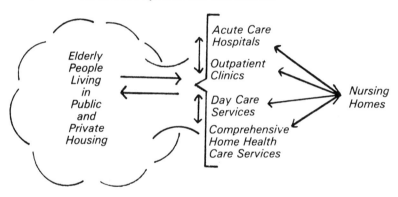

———⟶ = Orderly movement of older people to and from society and among facilities and services

A Simplified Health Care System for Older People

Recommended Changes

When implemented, the following recommendations will minimize deprivations and create an environment conducive to the satisfaction of patients' basic human needs.

Eliminate the Level of Care System

The level of care system is detrimental to the health and welfare of patients. It is abusive and causes unnecessary human hardships and displacements. Manipulation of categorizing criteria by hospital and nursing home personnel, and contrived diagnoses by physicians bring about assignments to preselected levels of care. This practice negates the intent of the system. The resultant uprootings violate human feelings, cause anxiety and stress, and adversely affect the mental and physical well-being of many people living in homes.

Change the Certificate-of-Need Laws

The certificate-of-need laws should allow for five empty beds for every 100 beds that are in demand. This will stimulate homes to compete for patients by providing a better quality of care.

This law should also allow for over-construction of homes in communities where substandard facilities exist and where substandard care is delivered. This can be determined by state public health inspection documentation. Such a regulation will support and foster quality care.

Eliminate Level of Care Utilization Review Committees in Nursing Homes

These committees, established to monitor level of care assignments and the need for nursing home care, are a farce. They waste the taxpayers' money, complicate the lives of patients, and create superfluous work and records. The truth is that there is only one consideration to be made when a patient is evaluated for care—does he or does he not need 24-hour nursing home services? A committee is not needed to make this determination, which is best made by the servicing physician who knows his client's history and family circumstances.

Require a Minimum of Four Hours of Nursing Time per Day per Patient for All Nursing Homes

This ratio would support good nurse coverage for the patients on all shifts. The common staffing pattern of two hours per patient does not permit time for the nursing staff to concern themselves with many of the patients' needs.

Recognize Nursing Home Patients' Basic Human Needs by Regulation

Servicing the needs documented in this book should be mandated by state regulation. State health inspectors should monitor conditions in the homes to assess whether or not the patients' basic human needs are being satisfied to a reasonable degree. For example, if patients have only meager possessions, if privacy is not allowed, if freedoms are limited, and if families do not visit some patients, then the home should be notified and alerted. These determinations can be made by inspector interviews with a limited number of patients and staff members. If the architectural design of the facility will not permit satisfaction of these needs, it should be so noted and the need for any related corrective action temporarily waived. This procedure would demonstrate a concern for patients' quality of life. It would also, in an indirect way, encourage architects to design more appropriate nursing homes.

Require All City, Town, and County Boards of Health to Inspect the Housekeeping Conditions and Sanitation Procedures Employed in All Nursing Homes Located in Their Communities

Local board of health inspectors should make quarterly inspections in nursing homes to monitor odor and sanitation conditions. They should be concerned for the frequency of cleaning, the number of personnel employed, the kinds of cleaning chemicals used, and the cleaning procedures involved. They should be equipped to demonstrate, counsel, and advise homes as to the kinds of cleaning agents they should use and how they should be applied. In addition, they should run infectious bacteria tests on the floors, windowsills, over-the-bed tables, chairs, and other objects that come in contact with patients.

Public Health Operating Standards Should Make Special Provisions for Rational Patients

Intermixing rational and disturbed patients should be disallowed as much as the design of the facility will permit. Having a mentally alert patient living in the same room with a disturbed patient should be prevented even if it means that bed vacancies will occur.

Develop New Federal and State Nursing Home Construction Standards Which Will Result in Homes Having Homelike Environments

Nursing home environments should emulate residential-style living and not hospital-style living. Homes that have copied acute care facility designs discourage the people residing in them from maintaining their individualities or satisfying many of their basic human needs. Innovative architecture formulated on the basis of those needs can help to foster individuality.

Eighty percent of the beds in newly constructed homes should be in private rooms. Existing homes which need renovation should plan to increase the number of private rooms to at least 50 percent. This is recommended to satisfy patients' needs for privacy and possessions. These rooms should be large enough to permit the occupants to use some of their own furniture. This includes dressers, bureaus, chairs, desks, other suitable items, and, under some circumstances, their own beds.

Creating a Human Services Department

The merit of organizing nursing homes like hospitals has not been questioned over the years even though the objectives of these two kinds of facilities differ. That is to say, hospitals seek cures whereas homes are not only concerned with the medical aspect of care but, most importantly, with giving patients a good quality of life.

The traditional way of delegating authority and assigning work duties in a nursing home fixes most of the responsibility for patient care on professional nurses. They are the overseers of all the procedures directly affecting the well-being of the patients. They have accountability above and beyond their medical duties and formal training. The director of nurses, in particular, is burdened with the responsibility of ensuring that all the patients' needs—medical *and* nonmedical—are met.

The consequence of organizing nursing homes like hospitals is that the nurses are not able to concentrate on the medical duties for which they were trained and educated. They must divide their time between skilled technical nursing and nontechnical responsibilities. The patients are dependent upon them for the satisfaction of all of their needs.

The creation of a new department within the nursing home environment called the *Human Services Department,* which would be responsible for the patients' personal care, should be considered. Heading this department would be a person with the title of *patient services director,* or other suitable designation.

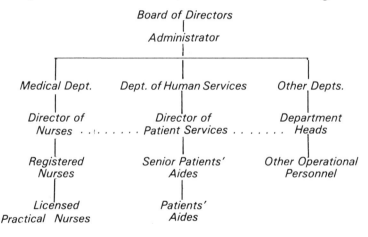

Key:

.... = Consultant advisory relationship
_____ = Direct authority relationship

Note: There are many considerations to be taken under advisement before instituting this kind of an organizational structure. The size of the facility affects the circumstances under which this would be implemented. Patients in larger homes, which have more difficult operational control problems, would benefit greatly from this type of system.

A Simplified Organizational Chart Showing the Position of the Patient Services Director

This person would supervise the nurses' aides who, with the new title of *patients' aides*, would continue to provide personal care to the patients and to respond to their nonmedical needs. The patient services director would report directly to the administrator and have equal status with the director of nurses. A consultant-advisory relationship would exist among the patient services director, the director of nurses, and each of the other department heads. It might be best if the educational requirements for this new director called for registered nurse training, but that is not absolutely necessary. A person exhibiting compassion and concern for nursing home patients would possess the most essential quality. A simplified organizational chart, graphically explaining this unique organizational structure, is shown in the diagram on the previous page.

The advantages of this kind of an organization are many, but there are two major ones. First, the professional nurses would be able to function at a maximum level and give the patients more concentrated skilled medical attention. Second, the patients' social, psychological, environmental, and other nonmedical basic human needs would get equal attention. The following list shows some of the basic responsibilities of the director of patient services.

1. To train patient aides.
2. To develop inservice training programs for aides and other nursing home personnel.
3. To supervise the patients' aides.
4. To supervise bed making.
5. To supervise patients' bathing procedures.
6. To supervise the delivery of all patient personal care.
7. To work closely with the heads of the other departments.
8. To encourage independence in patients.
9. To develop appropriate feeding procedures.
10. To facilitate patients' communication potential.
11. To encourage aides to become involved in the daily lives of patients.

12. To encourage visits from patients' families and friends.
13. To perfect systems which facilitate the movement of patients to recreational programs and other activities.
14. To perfect patients' exercise programs.
15. To research ways to satisfy all patients' basic nonmedical human needs.

Some Nursing Home Plan Ideas

The following sketches are presented to demonstrate that nursing homes can be different and innovative. They were developed after considering all of the basic human needs discussed in this book.*

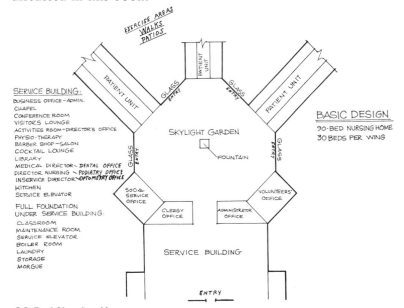

90-Bed Nursing Home

*These sketches have not been endorsed by a professional architect nor do they consider construction costs. Before any part of them is used to develop authentic plans, the nursing home construction regulations applicable to the state where they are to be used should be consulted.

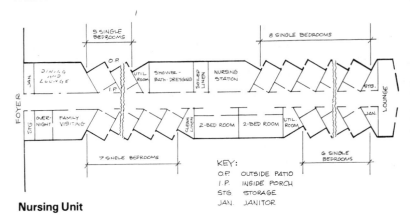

Nursing Unit

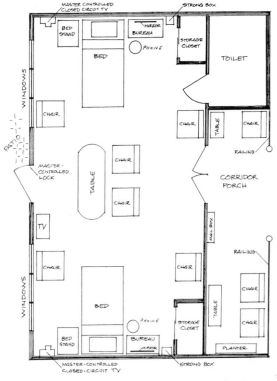

KEY: 225 SQ. FT. PER BED

Two-Bed Room

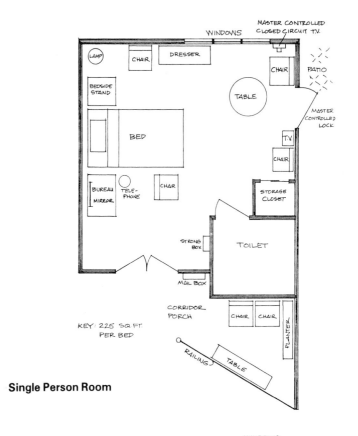

Single Person Room

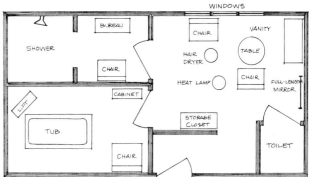

Bathing and Dressing Rooms

Some Nursing Home Design Specifications

The following design specifications have also been developed to satisfy the basic human needs of patients. They offer ideas to developers who wish to build innovative nursing homes. They were all considered when creating the facility sketches presented.

1. A minimum of 225 square feet of floor space per bed.
2. Individual four-drawer bureau for each patient.
3. Three armchairs with table and/or desk for each patient in every room.
4. Provision for television and telephone in each room.
5. Clothes closet: minimum size six feet high by 30 inches deep by five feet wide; with optional locking doors.
6. Each room to have a private toilet with a small vanity for personal care items; minimum 48 square feet; with hand bars.
7. One special family room in each unit for family visits and overnight stays; equipped with convertible sofa, tables, chairs, lamps, and other suitable furniture.
8. Picnic tables and fireplaces on the grounds.
9. Exercise area on the grounds complete with paved walkways for strolls and wheelchairs.
10. Each patient's room with a door leading to the outside (optional). This door to have a centrally controlled locking device.
11. Patio outside each patient's room (optional) or two patios for each unit.
12. Lawn furniture for the patios.
13. Each unit to have a minimum of two sitting rooms plus one family room and one room for congregate dining.
14. All doors leading to the outside to be locked with master-control for security purposes during certain hours.
15. Main entrance doors to have centrally controlled television monitoring of people entering the building.

16. At least one outside door of the facility which will be convenient for patients; to be opened by centrally controlled electric eye.
17. Provision for television monitoring of each patient bed. The cameras or lenses to be removable and activated only on permission of the patients and/or their families. To be centrally monitored and controlled.
18. Innovative shower and bathing section in each unit. This section to have the following:

> Separate dressing and undressing room, furnished with dresser and mirror, situated adjacent to the shower and bathing facilities.
> Separate bathtub room, minimum 100 square feet.
> Separate shower room, minimum 100 square feet.
> Appropriate home-like decor.

19. Carpeting permitted in visitor foyer at main entrance only.
20. Valuables box with locking device built into wall for each patient in every room.
21. Classroom for staff education programs. Large enough to service a number of staff equal to the number of beds in the facility.
22. Multiuse auditorium suitable for conversion to an ecumenical chapel.
23. Mailbox for receiving mail affixed to wall outside every room for each patient.
24. A main mailbox for outgoing mail in each unit.
25. Play area, with swings, on grounds for children.

An innovative facility such as has been described here might be called a "residential nursing home," since it is intended to be a home-like residence, a place where older human beings can live peacefully, can be creative if they wish, and are able to satisfy their needs and receive professional nursing supervision and care.

Index